Volunteers in hospice and palliative care

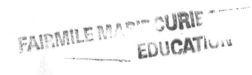

Volunteers in hospice and palliative care

A handbook for Volunteer Service Managers

Edited by

Derek Doyle

With a Foreword by

Dame Cicely Saunders

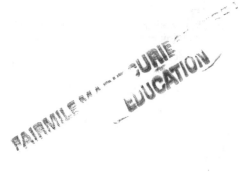

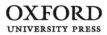

OXFORD
UNIVERSITY PRESS

OXFORD

UNIVERSITY PRESS

Great Clarendon Street, Oxford OX2 6DP

Oxford University Press is a department of the University of Oxford.
It furthers the University's objective of excellence in research, scholarship,
and education by publishing worldwide in

Oxford New York

Auckland Cape Town Dar es Salaam Hong Kong Karachi Kuala Lumpur
Madrid Melbourne Mexico City Nairobi New Delhi Shanghai Taipei Toronto

With offices in

Argentina Austria Brazil Chile Czech Republic France Greece
Guatemala Hungary Italy Japan South Korea Poland Portugal
Singapore Switzerland Thailand Turkey Ukraine Vietnam

Oxford is a registered trade mark of Oxford University Press
in the UK and in certain other countries

Published in the United States
by Oxford University Press Inc., New York

© Oxford University Press

The moral rights of the author have been asserted

Database right Oxford University Press (maker)

First published 2002

British Library Cataloguing in Publication Data

Data available

Library of Congress Cataloging in Publication Data (available)

ISBN 0 19 851608 8

Printed and bound in Great Britain
by Biddles Ltd., King's Lynn, Norfolk

Contents

Foreword

Roget's Thesaurus of English words and phrases lists under the heading 'Willingness', words that describe the attitudes and attributes of the volunteers who make up such an important part of the hospice team. These include: choice, spontaneity, aptitude, promptness, dedication, and loyalty. It also includes some warnings about a 'willing horse' or one who can become over involved as a 'do gooder', or of someone of whom others may easily take advantage.

These are all indications of the value of such work and also point out the need for careful selection, training, and management of volunteers if all involved are to achieve their true potential.

I met those talents in Lilian Pipkin, the Matron of St. Luke's Hospital, London (founded in 1893 as a Home for the Dying Poor) at which I myself was a volunteer. It had adapted itself over the years to one of the few 'hospices' to which, as a medical social worker, I was helping to transfer patients for end of life care in the late 1940s. My contact with the dying Jew David Tasma early in 1948 confirmed my desire to work in this field and, following his death, I offered to work there in the evenings as a Registered Nurse. Lilian Pipkin, was a remarkable woman, managing this small hospital of 48 beds for patients with advanced malignant disease with meagre resources, a hardworking but limited staff and one Red Cross volunteer. A very practical member of the Salvation Army, she discussed my aim to learn more of the excellent pain control I had observed on earlier visits and my need to verify my belief that I had a vocation in this field. She took time to describe the demands and rewards of such work, encouraged me to read some of the inspiring early reports of the Founder, Dr Howard Barrett, and sent me away to consider whether I could give loyalty as well as enthusiasm. When I returned to offer a weekly evening session, she took me on with a willingness to continue discussion of what the work really entailed. After a short time, I found myself in charge of a ward with the evening drug round as part of my commitment. It was in this volunteer role that I encountered the regular giving of four hourly oral morphine, which I later introduced and researched in St. Joseph's Hospice from 1958 and which has become the hallmark of the treatment of chronic and terminal pain.

Miss Pipkin was a model manager of volunteers as well as staff and, when St. Christopher's Hospice opened in 1967, she came to share some of her wisdom with the staff as it built up its own nursing and volunteer team.

In 1963, on an eight week tour of the United States, I spent time with the Director of Voluntary Services in a New York Cancer Hospital. She had founded and managed her team for ten years, stepping into the tradition which dates to at least the First World War and, historically, to all the wives and sweethearts who followed armies in order to care for the wounded as well, of course, as the Red Cross, which began working in the USA from 1881.

There were volunteers of all ages working throughout the hospital, offering many hours of regular and reliable service. I sensed that the department was a potent source of the positive atmosphere of that hospital and it inspired me with its competent compassion.

St. Christopher's Hospice appointed its own Volunteer Organizer among the first group of staff before it opened in 1967. We selected someone who lived locally, had a wide network of friends and contacts, a professional although unrelated background, and was a perceptive talent spotter. Allocated an office where the nearby room could be used by the ward volunteers for changing, she set up selection, training (involving a retired Sister Tutor, herself a volunteer), and ongoing regular support of her growing team with enduring vitality. The 16th Volunteer Organizer to be appointed in UK hospitals and the pioneer in the first modern hospice, she established the principles that have since been interpreted in many different cultures and with widely varied resources. Some teams have begun with nurses, doctors, social workers, chaplains, and others offering their spare time long before salaried posts became possible. Others give time as students when, as one said to me, 'I had nothing to offer but myself'. Many young volunteers receive inspiration for their futures from such work.

This brief history resonates in my mind with the characteristics of a visionary company as described in a book by Arie de Gens[1]. He portrays a successful company as one sensitive to its environment, with a sense of strong identity, tolerant of experiment (even eccentricity) with a readiness to adapt, while maintaining a deeply felt corporate pride. Such companies endure where others fail. Volunteers, unlike the salaried staff to which he refers, have a unique contribution to give to the developing, adapting life of a hospice team. Like them, they need open-hearted, sensitive and competent management if their motivation is to lead on to faithful service as they bring their life's experience to the help of others. This is so well illustrated in this volume.

Cicely Saunders
Founder/President
St. Christopher's Hospice, London

Reference

1. Arie de Gens (1999) *The Living Company*. Nicholas Brealey Publishing, London.

Preface

One of the most remarkable phenomena of the late 20th and early 21st century has been the development of 'hospice care' or, to give it its more descriptive title and the one preferred by health care professionals—'palliative care'. In our Introduction we have tried to describe this phenomenon and some of the many ways in which it is developing.

One feature of palliative care services is common to almost all models in whatever country they are operating. They use volunteers for a variety of roles, volunteers who need to be organized and led. This book is for them—the organizers of volunteers but, as we shall shortly explain, there are more appropriate terms for describing such individuals.

It is difficult to overstate the importance of volunteers in this remarkable occupation. They complement the work of the salaried professionals alongside whom they work in wards, clinics, day units, and bereavement services. In addition, they are to be found in coffee bars, charity shops, car services, libraries; arranging flowers, running creches for children of the staff and visitors, sitting with patients, reading to them—the list seems endless. More important than such a list of their roles is the contribution they make to the ambience, the atmosphere of the palliative care unit. They contribute to the 'homeliness' so often described by patients and visitors alike. They help to create what so many patients describe as that 'safe' feeling when you enter a hospice, that friendliness, informality, and genuine concern for people's needs that characterize such places. To a very large extent this remarkable contribution is made possible by the way they are selected, trained, supported, supervised, and managed by their leader, whatever such an invaluable person is termed.

Traditionally, the leader of the volunteers in a hospice was called the *Volunteer Co-ordinator*. The term reflected the important role of organizing what, in many hospices, was a veritable army of many hundreds of volunteers. In recent years, however, it has been appreciated that a better term is needed, one that truly describes both the role and the professional, paid nature of the job. For that reason in this book we have chosen to write about the *Volunteer Service Manager—VSM*. If the reader comes across the older term we have overlooked we crave their indulgence.

The publishers and ourselves needed no persuasion that such a handbook was needed. The work of a VSM is not only onerous; it is complex and multifaceted. It needs considerable skill, many gifts, and a sensitive, informed understanding of all that is meant by hospice/palliative care. In its scale it equals that of most other senior members of staff yet, we are informed, some VSMs are neither members of the senior management team nor is their work fully understood and appreciated by management and trustees.

We are very conscious that some readers will find nothing new in these pages. Others may feel overwhelmed with some of our suggestions and guidance, feeling that their unit and its volunteer team are too small to need such advice. However, it is hoped most will find something that challenges them, something they had never thought of, something they would like to try, something that reassures them or reaffirms what they have long been doing.

We hope that those working in small units will be fascinated by the chapters based on large, world-famous teaching hospitals, as well as on unique community palliative care services in one of the most needy parts of the world. We all have much to learn from them..

A few words about the style of the book. Each chapter stands alone and can be read on its own although, of course, we have cross-referenced to help our readers. We have chosen to use English as in the Oxford Dictionaries and trust our North American readers will not be offended. In many chapters, the authors, encouraged by the editor to do so, have made liberal use of bullet points in the hope that this will help readers to prioritize issues and facilitate referencing.

Readers will soon become aware of repetitions and apparent inconsistencies. The former remind us that some things are worth saying more than once, especially when expressed by people as experienced as our contributors. With all that experience they have inevitably developed different opinions, and different approaches and solutions to problems, hence the apparent inconsistencies in the book. Indeed, readers will be interested to read of some units using volunteers to provide 'hands-on' patient care and volunteers in many others never being in direct contact with patients.

We would stress that this is not a 'How to do it' book. Nothing here is immutable. There are other, possibly better, ways of tackling some of the issues we address. We offer the book to colleagues and friends worldwide as a handbook, not as a textbook, to help them in what we know well is a difficult, demanding, but always rewarding job.

It is a pleasure for me, as editor, to thank the contributors. It has been a genuine pleasure working with them, knowing that they wrote their chapters after long hard days of work, distilling many years of experience in hospice/palliative care. It also gives me pleasure to acknowledge the help and support I received from Ms Catherine Barnes, Commissioning Editor, and her staff at Oxford University Press.

May 2002   D. D

List of contributors

Dr Derek Doyle (Editor)
Hon. Vice President National Council for
Hospice and Specialist Palliative Care
Services
President Emeritus, the International
Association for Hospice and Palliative Care
Introduction

Dorothy Bates
Volunteer Service Manager
St. Michael's Hospice
Basingstoke
Hampshire, UK
**The managerial role of the Volunteer
Service Manager**

Kathleen Defilippi
Executive Director
South Coast Hospice
Port Shepstone
Kwa Zulu Natal
Republic of South Africa
**Volunteers Working in a community
palliative care service**

Erzsi Lyne de Ver
Formerly Volunteer and Personnel
Co-ordinator in a hospice; Presently
Management Consultant, York, UK
**The Position of the VSM within the
organization**

Nicola Grant
Volunteer Service Manager
Marie Curie Centre
Caterham, UK
Ethical issues for the VSM

Gill Hamilton
Formerly Volunteer Service Manager
St Columba's Hospice
Edinburgh, Scotland
**Legal issues for the VSM and the support
of volunteers**

Rosemary Hanley
Formerly Volunteer Service Manager
Austin and Repatriation Hospital
Heidelberg
Victoria, Australia
**Volunteers working in a comprehensive
palliative care service**

Mabuyi Mnguni
Deputy Director
South Coast Hospice
Port Shepstone
KwaZulu Natal
Republic of South Africa
**Volunteers working in a community
palliative care service**

Suzanne O'Brien
Co-ordinator
Hope and Cope
Jewish General Hospital
Montreal, Canada
**Volunteers working in a tertiary referral
teaching hospital**

Silke Lean
Volunteer Service Manager
Edenhall Marie Curie Centre
Hampstead, London, UK
**Health care professionals working as
volunteers**

Patricia McDermott
Volunteer Service Manager
Edenhall Marie Curie Centre
Hampstead, London
Professionals working as volunteers

Jenny Osterfield
Bereavement Service Co ordinator
St Michael's Hospice
Basingstoke
Hampshire, UK
Volunteers as bereavement counsellors

Ros Scott
Volunteer Service Manager
Rachel House
Kinross
Scotland, UK
Volunteers in a children's hospice

Sally-Ann Spencer-Gray
Lecturer in Palliative Care
The Education Department
Dove House Hospice
Hull, UK
The selection of volunteers and **The training and education of volunteers**

Ellen Wallace
Formerly Co-ordinator of Volunteers
Palliative Care Service
Royal Victoria Hospital
Montreal
Canada
Volunteers working in a tertiary referral teaching hospital

Chapter 1

Introduction

The evolution of hospice care

In many countries we have come to regard hospices as an accepted feature of our society, one which we almost take for granted, in much the same way as we expect every town to have its library, its swimming pool, and its civic centre. Most cities have at least one, its senior staff often affiliated with the local university. Most people know or have heard of someone who was cared for in a hospice. Friends and relatives are often serving as volunteers in their local hospice. Wherever we go we see collecting cans or read of fund-raising events—all for the local hospice.

It therefore comes as a surprise to many to learn that the first 'modern' hospice only opened in 1967. One has to speak of it in this way because, in the Middle Ages, there were hundreds of hospices, scattered along the trade and crusading routes of Europe, offering sustenance, care, and welcoming shelter to weary and often diseased and dying travellers. Most, if not all, were run by religious orders. Some remain to this day—wonderful museums to be visited and marvelled at with their airy rooms, drainage, and sanitation way ahead of their time, and facilities that must have had a wonderful effect on those who sought comfort and care within their walls.

In that relatively short time since 1967 hospices have sprung up all over the world so that as we write this book there are more than 6200 hospice services worldwide. What is important, however, is that word 'services'. No longer is a hospice always a building of bricks and mortar. It is, in a sense, a philosophy of care. There may indeed be a building for in-patients but equally hospice care may be given in a patient's home, in the wards of a general or a specialist hospital, in a nursing or residential home, or in a day care unit which the patient visits from home. Indeed, as needs have been identified it is now possible for those in prison to receive hospice care.

What is hospice care?

Whatever the place of care the overriding needs of the patient and the underpinning principles of their care are the same. The patients are all suffering from advanced life-threatening illness. They may have only months or even weeks of life left and what they need—and what the hospice is there to provide—is relief of their suffering whatever its cause, whatever its nature—whether it is physical, spiritual or emotional. Hospice care focuses on quality of life rather than length of life—neither abbreviating it nor trying to extend it artificially. Not only is hospice care about quality of life—it is equally about the value of the person's life and helping him or her to find meaning in life as it draws to a close. Finally, hospice care embraces respect for the suffering and the needs of relatives and close friends.

It might well be pointed out—as indeed it has often been—that such compassionate, holistic caring is surely the hallmark of all care given to patients whatever the illness or its stage and whoever is the carer, be it doctor, nurse, pastoral care worker or social worker. This emphasis on patient-centred care focusing on quality of life, patient autonomy, and profound respect for the individual should be an integral feature of all care. Sadly, however, that is not always the case.

In recent years with many new techniques and drugs making cure a possibility more effort has been spent on trying to cure than on providing care for those who cannot be cured. Increasingly, hospitals are assumed to be the best places for treatment and care when, in fact, evidence and experience show that most people with a terminal illness prefer to stay at home as long as possible, although not necessarily to die at home. Hospitals are certainly appreciated by people when they need highly specialized care, often enhanced by modern technology, but there comes a time when they want a less frenetic atmosphere, some peace and quiet to think and to enjoy time with loved ones. A hospice aims to provide that—an atmosphere tailored to the needs of the dying, a place where it is safe to laugh as well as to cry, where it is safe to 'be yourself' and, as so many people have said, a safe place to die, paradoxical as that may sound.

Why call it 'palliative care'?

In this very short space of time the word 'hospice' has been accepted into the English language and come to mean something very special to many people. They associate it with the care their loved ones and friends received when they needed it. They know of the warmth of its care, the dedication of its staff, the visits paid to people being looked after at home, and the creative vitality of day hospices where hobbies are developed, new skills discovered, and rich friendships formed. Why then was the term 'palliative care' ever coined and adopted? What was wrong with 'hospice'?

There are several reasons. The term was probably first attached to this philosophy of care in French Canada where the word 'hospice' means something quite different from what we have been describing. There and in many other parts of the world it was felt that a term was needed which described what happens in a 'hospice', a term which would be understood by doctors and nurses because it was part of their daily vocabulary. Such a word is 'palliative' which has long been used to describe comfort care when cure was impossible. Palliation might be easing pain when the underlying problem cannot be eradicated or relieving breathlessness, restoring appetite, helping sleep, or explaining what is happening to lessen the anxieties. It might simply mean being there when someone is lonely on what must surely be the loneliest journey any of us ever makes.

There is no difference between hospice and palliative care. Both describe the same thing but whereas 'hospice' is the word beloved of the public, 'palliative care' is the term now accepted and reasonably well understood by health care professionals the world over. All such care must, in popular jargon, be interdisciplinary or interprofessional. This means much more than doctors, nurses, social workers, and the professions allied to medicine all working for the common good of the patient ('multiprofessional'). It means that they share a common goal for each patient under their care; that they know the skills and gifts each can bring to that care; that they share their skills and their insights so that the care they give as a team is better than could come from any one individual; and that they support each other. The analogy with a sports team is obvious—all working together, as equals, for a common goal.

When we refer to the work of the team we speak of *palliative care.* When we speak of what doctors do as part of that team we use the term *palliative medicine* and when speaking of the work of the nurses it is *palliative nursing.* This clearer definition of what everyone does, together with the vast increase in knowledge and expertise in recent years has brought about the recognition of both palliative medicine and palliative nursing as specialties, first in the UK, then in Australia, New Zealand, Hong Kong, Sweden, Romania, and Poland.

Education and training in palliative care

It has long been recognized by many health care professionals that they need better education and training in this field of care than they ever received in the past. Who better to contribute to that than those working in palliative care, particularly when they have devoted many years to advanced training to qualify as specialists? For that reason most hospices/palliative care services have medical and nursing students to visit the units, release their senior staff to lecture in the universities and colleges of nursing, and have education departments visited by literally thousands of people each year. All of this is essential but it imposes on the staff a responsibility to see that so many professional visitors do not damage the ambience being created for the patients, or infringe their privacy and dignity.

Palliative care services

We have already seen that hospice/palliative care need not mean an *in-patient unit* like a mini-hospital though such units continue to be built and developed around the world. In the UK, four-fifths of them are detached from any hospital and very largely dependent on the generosity of the general public. The other one-fifth are in, or within the grounds of, National Health Service hospitals and run as part of that hospital. Busy as they always are, in fact only a small percentage of people dying with diseases, such as cancer, actually die in an in-patient palliative care unit.

Most people have their initial investigations, are diagnosed, then given their active treatment and often keep being readmitted to general and specialist hospitals until they die. The challenge was therefore how to help them, how to offer them the highest standard of palliative care without them having to move to another place such as the district hospice/palliative care unit. The answer lay in forming *hospital palliative care teams*, based in secondary and tertiary referral hospitals. They could see patients with advanced illness in wards familiar to them from previous admissions, advise on appropriate care and, in so doing, enable young hospital doctors and nurses to see how effective such expert palliative care can be. Today, hospital palliative care teams are the fastest growth areas in this subject, to be found not only in every cancer centre but in many large, even world-famous hospitals in the UK, Canada, USA and Australasia.

As we have said, many people when they sense or have had it confirmed that their illness is far advanced, ask to stay at home provided their loved ones, assisted by the family doctor and community nurses, will be able to look after them. To enable that to happen *community palliative care services* were created and are now to be found, in their thousands, around the world. Patients are visited at home, their needs are assessed, and advice given to them, their lay carers and to their professional carers. After that they continue to be visited, sometimes being brought in to *day hospice*, sometimes helped in their visits to hospital and some-times offered a bed in the in-patient unit for terminal care, for control of their symptoms or as a respite for their relatives.

Most community palliative care teams are advisory as described but a few teams offer comprehensive care in the home. They take out beds, equipment, medica-tions, carry out minor surgical procedures if they will ease the patient's suffering, and even offer round-the-clock nursing. Increasingly, as will be described in this book, they are to be found where resources are scanty, doctors and nurses are scarce, and drugs not available.

Day hospices have just been mentioned. Patients are brought in from home by volunteer transport once or twice a week. After a cup of coffee and a chat they busy themselves with whatever activity or craft is assigned to them by the occupational therapist who has assessed their needs. It might be a long-standing hobby or interest like woodwork or painting, or a new one such as pottery, enamel work or indoor gardening. After lunch (usually with 'just a little drink') there may be entertainment laid on, or the visit of a famous actor or sports person, until mid-afternoon when they are taken back home, usually tired but delighted to have been with others in the same boat as themselves and surprised at how much they managed to do.

Of course, not all palliative care services offer all that we have described here. Those that do, however, we might term *comprehensive palliative care services*. In addition to the in-patient unit with anything from six to more than one hundred beds, there will also be a community palliative care service, a day hospice/palliative care unit, even a hospital palliative care team, a bereavement service, and an education and training programme.

Clearly, there is no right model and no wrong model. A small hospice/palliative care unit with a few beds may be exactly what a small community needs whereas somewhere else the need is more for assistance in keeping people at home or giving respite care. What matters is that the needs of the community—be it a small town or a suburb of a major city—are thoroughly assessed before any palliative care programme is planned and then the most appropriate model established to meet those needs. Sadly, this seldom happens and in some places there has been over-provision of some palliative care models and even unhealthy competition between providers.

Who are the patients?

Professionals working in this field of palliative care have, as you would expect, devised various working definitions of their work and described the patients they are qualified to care for. Basically, it is people with far-advanced, life-threatening illness for whom cure is not possible and for whom the focus of care must be their quality of life.

For many years, almost everyone who was referred by his/her doctor for palliative care had a malignant disease, usually cancer. Experience had taught us that they often suffered not only appalling pain but also loss of appetite, nausea, sickness, increasing frailty, and weight loss, all of which could be helped with skilled palliation.

Gradually, it came to be recognized that the same principles could be applied to many other, non-malignant conditions, such as heart disease, respiratory problems, advanced endocrine disorders, and neurological problems, such as muscular dystrophy, motor neurone disease, and multiple sclerosis. Today, palliative care also plays a major part in the care of people with HIV and AIDS. Indeed, in several cities special AIDS hospices have been established and many community palliative care services are exclusively for AIDS patients.

In the adult hospices a high percentage of the patients are admitted for terminal care although, of course, they may have been under the community palliative care service for many months and also attending the day hospice. Children's hospices are different. Few of the children are admitted for terminal care and most are there, as is explained in Chapter 10, to give a welcome and much-needed respite to the parents. Many of them have congenital conditions, often quite rare, and are heavily dependent on loving carers in their homes.

The workload of hospice/palliative care services

The popular notion of a hospice is a place of great tranquillity, its staff spending most of the time sitting quietly by the bedsides, admitting a new patient every few days, few, if any, of the patients ever able to return home but happy to be there until they die. In fact, such places are extremely busy.

The average length of time people are in a hospice/palliative care unit is usually less than two weeks. Between 40% and 60% are discharged home into the care of their family doctor and the community palliative care service. Most units, depending on the number of beds they have, admit between 500 and 1000 patients each year. At any one time between 100 and 300 will be under care in their own homes. Whereas until a very short time ago almost every patient had a form of cancer, today 20% to 30% will have some other life-threatening illness.

The professional staff

The so-called specialist palliative care services have senior staff—physicians and nurses—who are all accredited specialists. To obtain that honour they have had to train for at least eight to ten years after qualifying as doctors or registered nurses. Supporting them are the 'professions allied to medicine' (PAMs) which include the physiotherapists, occupational therapists, music and art therapists, dieticians, and nutritionists. Larger units also have at least one social worker, a pastoral care worker (chaplain), clinical pharmacist, and if they are fortunate, a clinical psychologist.

The larger hospice/palliative care units have a library with its own librarian, often serving as a resource for local universities and colleges. The educational work of the unit is led by a full-time lecturer/educationalist often assisted by other lecturers. Some of the teaching is, of course, done by other members of the clinical staff.

Supporting them all is the administrative staff under a Chief Executive responsible for the overall management, fund-raising, all staff matters, and public relations.

If there is one word which should, and indeed nearly always does, describe the work of a hospice/palliative care service it is *professionalism*. Each member of staff is carefully selected, given excellent pre-service and in-service training and supervision, is well supported, and sets the highest standards for their work, their loyalty, their work relationships, whatever their role or position within the unit and its many diverse services.

The volunteers

'Professionalism' may be the word that best describes the work but ask patients and their relatives what words they would use to describe their impressions of a hospice or a palliative care unit or community service and they will say 'homely, friendly, relaxed, safe, unthreatening'. They will describe how they were always made welcome, were helped by people who were 'approachable, understanding, ready to listen, and who knew what was needed'.

Why do people use these terms and say that hospices are different from most hospitals? After all, both have skilled professionals, all dedicated to the good of their patients.

It can only be due to an unusual wedding of two groups—the professional staff of doctors, nurses, chaplains, and many others, and the army of volunteers. Just how this army is recruited, trained, supervised, and supported, how its members are helped to work side-by-side with the professional team, and who leads this army—this is the story of this book.

Volunteers are so much a feature of this work that we are in danger of taking them for granted. Not only that. We can overlook the skills needed by the person who manages the volunteer service, whether that person is termed the 'Co-ordinator of

Volunteers' or, much more preferable, the 'Volunteer Service Manager—VSM'. This book is for them, whatever their title or job description.

Their work is difficult, always challenging, always varied and often deeply rewarding. It calls for imagination and vision, infinite patience and consummate skills of diplomacy as well as sensitive understanding of people. It calls for managerial, organizational, and leadership skills and an informed and profound understanding of hospice and palliative care, how it is provided and who its patients and providers are.

This little book has been written for them—the managers of volunteer services throughout this exciting world of hospice and palliative care.

Why this book is needed

There are many parallels between the professional ('paid') staff and the volunteers. For example, it used to be thought that any doctor or nurse could look after a person with a terminal illness—it was thought to be something that came naturally, like breathing or eating. It did not require any thought. No training was needed for it! How wrong we were. It was because of these misunderstandings that so many patients suffered as they did. Experience has shown that to do this work properly, as it deserves, and as our patients have every right to expect requires not only training, but also careful selection, inspired leadership, and understanding support. The same applies to volunteers.

Doctors and nurses need inspired, informed leadership. So do volunteers. They both need someone who knows about their work, knows its challenges as well as its rewards; someone who knows how to get the best out of them and bring about genuine job satisfaction.

Professional staff need to be supported—and to feel supported—in their day-to-day work. So do volunteers. Neither group seeks sympathy or praise but they both need to know there is someone who understands how stressed they can sometimes feel, how disappointed, how frustrated.

Both professionals and volunteers like to feel that they are working in a well-organized, well-managed organization—a 'business-like one' with clear channels of communication, well-planned budgets, and well-informed senior management who appreciate what they do and who they are.

What are some of the features of a Volunteer Service Manager's job?

How curious that people ever thought *anyone* could manage a volunteer service. All they needed was some spare time, a charming manner, a clutch of social graces, and the gift of persuasion! Not surprisingly, experience has shown that the challenge is great and to do justice to the job it requires a special kind of person. This book looks at the work of the Manager/Co-ordinator of Volunteers and sets out how to ensure that it is characterized by as high a degree of professionalism as that of any of the salaried staff.

The writer once attended a lecture about the gifts and attributes a manager of a volunteer service needed to do bring to the job. In preparation, the speaker had asked volunteers, professional staff, and even patients and relatives what they thought. She then flashed on to the screen dozens of words they had come up with—diplomacy, tact, vision, understanding of people, knowledge of palliative care, office skills, public relations skills, public speaking skills, knowledge of employment law, understanding of ethics, interviewing skills...The list seemed endless but perhaps it was all summed up in the final quote—'She needs to be like a God but never behave like one!'

In this book, we shall address many of the responsibilities of VSMs. How do you go about recruiting and selecting, training, and supporting volunteers? How do you interview and how do you reject someone? How do you select for different roles—a vacancy in the day hospice, another one in the flower arranging team, and several in the charity shops?

What management and office skills and experience does a VSM need? Is computer literacy necessary? When does efficiency become an intrusive obsession likely to annoy your volunteers? What records are essential and what are not essential but likely to be very useful in day-to-day management?

Is it asking too much that managers have an understanding of medical ethics? As every experienced co-ordinator will attest and every long-serving hospice professional confirm, there are occasions when confidentiality is breached without people recognizing what they have done. How easy it is to tell someone of a mutual friend you saw in the hospice when doing your voluntary work there—even that is breaching confidentiality. Would an understanding of the ethics of resource allocation be helpful or an informed understanding of the issues surrounding voluntary euthanasia and physician-assisted suicide?

Are there legal issues any manager needs to be conversant with? Clearly, laws differ from one country to another and this little book has been prepared for colleagues worldwide but certain issues are shared by all. Do volunteer drivers need a special insurance policy? Who is responsible if a patient is allowed to fall out of a wheel chair being pushed by a volunteer or slips when being assisted to walk to the toilet?

This raises even bigger questions. Should volunteers ever give 'hands-on' patient care? If so, is it to save the salary of a qualified nurse or to release a nurse to do something 'more important'? Even this question leads to an even more basic one. Why do we have volunteers at all? Is it to make the place more user-friendly, more like home? Is it to save money or to do tasks modern nurses do not like doing? Is it possible to have too many volunteers around the place? Are there some tasks that volunteers should never be asked or expected to do?

As paediatricians remind us, children are not miniature adults. They differ in very many respects. Are children's hospices just adult hospices painted and equipped for little people? Could a person be equally effective and valued as a volunteer in a children's hospice as in the adult hospice down the road where they have worked for several years? This and many other issues are addressed in Chapter 10, which is devoted to children's hospices.

Are the principles and the problems the same whether you are a volunteer in a 10-bed hospice or working as part of a hospital palliative care team in a 1000-bed hospital? Are things different in Australia and North America? If you are a volunteer in a deprived, AIDS-ridden part of Africa is it reasonable that you should get some very modest payment for your work or is that changing your status from a volunteer to a member of the paid staff? This too will be addressed in the book.

Research has shown that well-trained, well-supervised volunteers are as effective at bereavement support as professional counsellors. Who is suitable for this work and how can they be trained, supervised, and supported? Should this be yet another responsibility of the VSM and if not, whose should it be?

As readers will have observed, until now we have spoken as though all volunteers are untrained people, with hearts of gold and with some time to spare to help those less fortunate than themselves. However, there are others who offer their services. These are the highly trained health care professionals like doctors, nurses, physiotherapists, and occupational therapists, and, an increasingly common event in modern hospice care—those who have trained in some branch of complementary or alternative medicine. What should be the relationship of the manager with them? Should they be accountable to manager or to the senior physician or director of nursing? What are the legal aspects of 'employing' them?

No, being a manager of a volunteer service is not the easy task some people have thought it to be. We hope this book will bring clarity to it for some, will smooth the way for others and help everyone to get even greater satisfaction out of doing it.

Professionalism must be the keyword.

Chapter 2

The managerial role of the Volunteer Service Manager

Volunteer co-ordinators in the majority of palliative care units are required to act as managers and are gradually being recognized as Voluntary Service Managers.[1] There is some debate about the relevant models of management appropriate for working with volunteers. The conclusion is perhaps not so much that one model is more appropriate than another but more about finding a management style 'in keeping with the values and ethos of voluntary action'.[2]

This chapter sets out to explain the diverse role of the Voluntary Service Manager (VSM) promoting the idea that the person appointed to such a post, in whatever size of organization, should have the experience and calibre to reflect the responsibilities involved. Frequently, organizations are tempted to appoint a less able person because it is assumed that to 'organize' volunteers who are freely giving of their time, is easier than managing staff. In so doing, organizations can enter in to a circle of ineffectuality, often resulting in an unhappy and unproductive volunteer 'workforce' and a negative approach throughout the organization to the benefits of working with volunteers.

So, what is it about the role that moves it from a co-ordinating role to one of management?

First, co-ordinating is one-dimensional, implying the organization of a group of like-minded individuals who all agree on a common task and the way to carry out that task. In hospices, volunteers, if managed effectively, can provide a vibrant, energized, and focused workforce, capable of contributing to and enhancing the quality of the care provided whilst also allowing the budget to be extended in imaginative and creative ways. Such a workforce is made up of a complex and diverse group of people. Diversity of people and tasks requires careful management.

Many small volunteer organizations are 'staffed' entirely by volunteers. What distinguishes hospices and other palliative care organizations from these is that the core of the service is provided by paid staff. While volunteers often outnumber the staff and in some cases might be seen as a threat, staff and volunteers are required to work alongside and support each other in what is often a fragile and highly charged atmosphere. It falls to the VSM to be responsible for good volunteer/staff relations and to facilitate an effective working relationship—a complex task!

The tasks and responsibilities carried out by volunteers do not exist in isolation to the working of the organization, and the scope and volume of these volunteer activities will vary depending on the organization's willingness to harness these skills together with the success and development of the organization itself. The reverse is also true particularly in palliative care where units have traditionally depended on the contribution made by the volunteer workforce.

Organizations, when planning future strategy, must consider any volunteer contribution anticipated alongside any resource implications. For example, in most day care services, volunteers play a large part, whether it is to drive, to offer diversional therapy, to make teas/coffees, etc. In planning to introduce or expand a day care service, it makes sense that the provider of these resources, the VSM, is involved at the strategic and early planning stages of such a project. Availability (or otherwise) of possible volunteers, training, and support costs all need to be taken into account but are frequently overlooked at the initial planning stage. Volunteers are not stored in cupboards waiting to be produced whenever needed at a moment's notice—a frequent misapprehension amongst paid staff!

Finally, in acknowledging that it is the VSM's responsibility to provide the equivalent of the 'human resources' function in recruiting, selecting, training, and supporting the organization's volunteers then here we complete the 'management portfolio' of the role.

Before examining this role in greater detail, it is important to clarify one other dimension, often misunderstood. The role cannot be to manage the volunteer work force *per se*, for it is widely accepted that no manager can effectively manage large numbers of people. Since many hospice volunteer workforces number in the hundreds, clearly this would be an impossible task. And so it is the volunteer *service* that is managed, and the direction of the volunteers themselves is devolved to department managers/team leaders just as in the case of paid staff.

In summary, the major role of the VSM is not to work directly with volunteers, except in their recruitment and selection, but to work with management on a strategic planning level, and individual staff to help them manage, train and retain their volunteers.

Working in palliative care

Many of the fundamental aspects of volunteer management in palliative care are the same as in any other organization but there are some specific elements that are important and which influence both the job content and the person specification for the role incumbent.

- The working environment has a high 'emotional' content which means that much more care has to be taken in the recruitment and selection of volunteers.
- It is vitally important that the VSM is personally emotionally strong and able to understand and support volunteers exposed to the sadness of loss and bereavement.

- VSMs should have a firm grasp of the philosophy underpinning the care given whether or not they themselves are from a health care background. In many hospices the VSM attends the weekly multidisciplinary review of patient care giving them a regular background and insight as well as contributing to discussions and planning for patients.

The management role

Planning for volunteers

In planning for a volunteer service the first task is to help the organization to focus on how it intends to relate to volunteers. The following fundamental questions must be considered and agreed:

- Why does the organization wish to involve volunteers? (Is it just because most other units have them or, as it needs to be, from a genuine belief that volunteers will truly bring benefits?)
- What are the organization's expectations of volunteers?
- Will the organization be prepared actively and openly to embrace the involvement of volunteers throughout the organization and to promote this among the staff?
- What resources is the organization prepared to devote to the development of a volunteer service?

Once these general principles have been agreed by the Board of Trustees down, there is in place a firm foundation for a successful volunteer service. Everyone in the organization then knows what to expect and what is expected of them and it is a powerful motivating force for volunteers, encouraging loyalty and commitment.

A similar exercise should be undertaken to define the aim and establish principles to underpin the work of the voluntary services department itself. For example an agreed aim might read:

> …to provide voluntary support for the organization, to contribute to the improved quality of life of patients and their carers, whilst enabling volunteers to achieve their individual potential and maximum satisfaction.[3]

Principal functions of the department might include:[3]

- Recruiting, selecting and placing suitable volunteers who will:
  - provide to patients and carers a service that complements that which is provided by the professional team, and
  - support other staff in the performance of their duties;
- assist staff in the implementation of policy and good practice in the day-to-day deployment of volunteers;
- develop the potential of the volunteer resource and encourage new initiatives to meet identified needs.

Other functions will complete the service that the department will perform on behalf of the organization. More detailed decisions on where volunteers work, what they do and how they do it become part of the ongoing management role of the VSM. These decisions should all be based on written policies and procedures,[3] covering areas, such as administrative and clinical procedures, strategies, and statistics, and review processes.

Strategic planning (see also Chapter 3)

As the organization develops and external circumstances change so emerges the role for the VSM to keep informed about the changing needs of both the organization and the wider world of palliative care. In order to support and contribute to the business planning of the organization, the VSM must maintain an awareness of wider external implications for volunteering. This includes such issues as the changing political climate, including government activities, policies and new legislation, local demographic trends, including an understanding of the local cultural environment where attitudes towards volunteering may be different, and the changing economic climate. Assuming that hospices will continue to depend on a significant contribution from volunteers, the trends in availability of volunteers as a resource will play a key part in future plans.

Budgeting for volunteers

Establishing a realistic budget, operating within it and reviewing performance before renegotiating a new budget creates an efficient and effective way to develop the volunteer service in line with the organization's working principles and priorities.

Costing

Some organizations make a mistake by believing that the introduction of volunteers is a cheap option with such low costs that no formal budgeting is necessary. It becomes clear how necessary it is to agree a budget, allocate resources, and effectively manage them by examining some of the possible costs of a volunteer service:

- Good volunteer practice in the UK,[4] based on equality of opportunity for all, encourages the reimbursement of expenses to all volunteers.
- Recruitment techniques such as advertising, leaflets, etc.
- Training and support for volunteers using facilitators, rooms, equipment, etc.
- Salary costs for the VSM together with their training and support.
- Insurance cover for the work of the volunteers.
- Other overhead costs. (The element often forgotten in the planning for volunteers is the allocation of such simple resources as—where will the person sit or will there be a spare computer available during the time the volunteer is on duty?)

A detailed costing exercise is thus the first important step of budget planning. The VSM will then discuss with the line manager (or Chief Executive, depending on the size of the organization) the allocation of appropriate resources.

Allocation of resources

The allocation of resources to the volunteer department should be no different than for any other department in the organization. It may be that all staff in small embryonic units combine forces to fund raise to obtain the wherewithal to operate. However, in larger and more established organizations funding needs to be organized through a central source not only to achieve control and consistency of resource allocation but also to avoid duplication of fund-raising activity and running the risk of creating fund-raising fatigue amongst possible donors. In any case, funding will probably come from a number of different sources and this income should form the basis of resources available to meet the organization's expenditure needs.

Budget setting

The agreed budget is usually set in advance on an annual basis with reviews carried out regularly during that time to monitor its effectiveness and to allow the readjustment of targets where this is possible. Most organizations will have their own timing and procedures for the management of budgets and so naturally the process for the volunteer department will form part of these. A VSM looking to acquire the appropriate knowledge base to participate in budget setting, should find it as part of any basic diploma-type management course, or as the basis for short one-off courses often run by local or national training agencies.

The personnel manager

Although managing volunteers does have some specific needs of its own there are certain principles of personnel management which serve the volunteer world well and require key skills from a VSM. In particular, this is the case in small organizations where no one specializes in the personnel function.

Recruitment and selection (see also Chapter 4)

Clearly, the VSM with no previous experience needs to acquire confidence in interviewing skills and should have access to a private room in which to meet potential volunteers.

One of the most difficult situations to handle in the selection process is 'saying no'. In palliative care it is sometimes not the right environment and so an offer of time and skills has to be turned down. Although it is occasionally possible to guide potential volunteers in another direction, it requires skilled handling on the part of the VSM to minimize the disappointment for the volunteer and at the same time to protect the reputation of the organization.

Training and support (see also Chapters 4 and 5)

Assessing training and support needs of volunteers and identifying how to meet them is done by the VSM in conjunction with each department concerned. A knowledge and understanding of this process is a key skill for a VSM to have or to acquire.

Although most training sessions will involve members of the professional team, some sessions, such as introducing new volunteers to the organization's policies and procedures, can be led by the skilled VSM. As well as being able to lead a training session, it is important that the VSM is at ease in facilitating groups since regular meetings of volunteer teams is a common way to offer ongoing regular support, an opportunity to address any issues of concern and to communicate information about organization developments and events.

Volunteers who are distressed or upset by their work for any reason need to know they can go to the VSM for support, particularly if they feel unable to talk to anyone else in the organization. The VSM needs to be familiar with basic counselling skills and be a good listener.

Motivation and retention

Hospices and other palliative care organizations will attract a significant number of volunteers in the first instance just because of their belief and support for the cause itself. At this point, understanding what brings someone to volunteer is a key aspect of the selection process as it may determine whether or not you, as the VSM, decide to accept this offer of help.

Since introducing a new volunteer to the organization and providing training is a fairly long process with a significant investment of time and resources, it becomes important to encourage good volunteers to stay. In the UK, increasing competition for a decreasing number of people prepared to volunteer[4] is another factor making it important to retain the volunteers already in place. Most volunteers will only do so if they are well motivated.

'In order to retain support—both as fund-raisers and as volunteers—hospices must ensure that volunteers are involved, understand and agree with the working practice of voluntary hospices'.[5] This was one of the findings of a survey, which produced other interesting conclusions about what volunteers look for from the hospices in which they work. A different survey reports: 'There is some evidence that the introduction of changes without consultation or discussion with volunteers may have had a negative effect upon the commitment, sense of belonging, and motivation of some long serving volunteers'.[6]

Ongoing training provides an opportunity to show that the organization values the work of the volunteers and the regular support of team meetings offers the chance to discuss issues of concern.

The role of the VSM here is not an easy one. Volunteers often feel very strongly about certain issues, sometimes with justification, sometimes not. For the VSM, deciding what to take further and what to challenge comes from knowing the organization, its people, its policies and procedures, and priorities. Volunteers need to trust the VSM and know their point of view will be heard and respected even if, in the end, it is impossible to meet their request. The ability to handle difficult situations is vital.

There are many other examples of difficult situations which a VSM must be skilled enough to handle. It may be from a volunteer becoming too old or unable to carry out duties safely, to volunteers who continually overstep boundaries, from a volunteer suffering a personal bereavement, to a conflict of opinion whether with staff or other volunteers. Negotiating between volunteers and staff requires a good deal of diplomacy and tact. The VSM needs to be readily accessible to both volunteers and staff in an effort to keep a finger 'on the pulse' and to address difficult situations before the need arises to resort to formal procedures.

There is some debate about whether the principles of appraisal and review could or should be applied to volunteers. Whilst acknowledging that some volunteers (e.g. those gaining experience for a future career) might welcome an in-depth appraisal with targets and learning objectives, it is important to remember that many volunteers do not want to be involved in such serious undertakings. This is a good example of needing to balance the good intention of the willing citizen with the developing professionalism of the world of volunteering. But volunteers do like to know if they are doing a good job or if they can do better, and they do ask for feedback. Taking time out with a volunteer to look at their contribution to the organization is a way of valuing them and can do much to both motivate and encourage a high quality of 'performance'. The best person to sit down with the volunteer is the leader of the team in which the volunteer works. The role of the VSM is to work with the team leader in setting these meetings up, supporting the team leader in carrying them out and monitoring the outcomes (see also Chapters 5 and 6).

There is little doubt that the subject of motivation is complex but it is an area where the VSM must have insight and knowledge if valued volunteers are to be encouraged to want to stay.

Legislation

People volunteer for many reasons and for most there is an element of altruism and citizenship involved. For some, their wish is 'to serve', for others, they strive to 'make a difference', both groups often driven by an idealistic zeal! It is easy under these circumstances for staff in organizations to overlook, and hard for some volunteers to accept, that not 'anything goes' and activities can be restricted by the bounds of the laws of the land. The VSM role is not only to ensure that good practice is followed but also a greater challenge is often in enabling the enthusiastic volunteer to understand the need to comply with the regulations.

Since it is normal practice for all volunteers to be covered by the organization's insurance policies, it is an important task for the VSM to ensure clarity of volunteer role definition as demanded by insurance companies, taking in to account a risk assessment of tasks to be undertaken.

Staff and volunteers working together

Paid staff can often feel threatened by the introduction of volunteers.[7] In order to help maximize the mutual benefits it is an important responsibility of the VSM to reassure staff about the place in the organization of the volunteers by providing a framework where the role and status is defined and understood. This could be presented visually by including the volunteer roles in the organization chart. In addition, staff job descriptions should include a paragraph on their responsibility towards volunteers.

When introducing a new volunteer project, the VSM can gain the confidence of staff members by involving them at every step of the way from the planning stage onwards. This approach has the advantage of encouraging staff to 'own' the project and to support it even through difficult times. In addition, asking team members to participate in the training of volunteers often eases their anxieties about how a project will work and the part the volunteers will play. It also gives an opportunity to the volunteers to explore their thoughts and ideas with the staff thus engendering an atmosphere of trust. However, while it is important that the VSM reinforces the positive message about working with volunteers, they must also be open and willing to hear any voices of concern, and work towards resolving any problems from any source.

Once volunteers are in place it is important to maintain liaison with the department head and review how the volunteer role is progressing as well as keeping lines of communication open with the volunteers. It should be clear to whom the volunteers are accountable and to whom they should go if there is a problem. The role of the VSM is to offer individual support to this member of staff and in addition may also provide written guidelines or training if it is felt necessary. Volunteers value feedback and the person in the role of supervisor should be helped to perform this role with each volunteer.

Often, the sheer numbers of volunteers working in a department together with frequent shift variations for staff make communication and supervision difficult. At the very least, there should be regular volunteer team meetings at which a member of the staff team is present. It may be appropriate to appoint key members of staff and/or volunteer team leaders to represent the views of both groups and thus develop a sharing of ideas and views.

Volunteer team leaders can also undertake other key roles and this concept is particularly beneficial in large organizations where often hundreds of volunteers are involved. It introduces another tier of responsibility and one that provides a more personal point of contact for a larger group of volunteers than is otherwise possible. These volunteer team leaders can, for example, also organize rotas and help with induction and training. They work closely with the VSM, reporting regularly, and are a vital link to the department in which their team works. Different hospices have different formulae which work for them. One working example is St. Columba's Hospice in Edinburgh.[8] One such model is shown in Figure 2.1.

Other staff team members should know the appropriate lines of responsibility and communication for volunteers and be encouraged to respect the volunteer role. It may also be useful to issue a set of guidelines to help them understand how to best work alongside their volunteer colleagues. When new staff join the organization it should be part of their induction programme to spend time with the VSM to help smooth the pathway towards working with volunteers.

Some simple features to encourage integration and a positive supportive atmosphere throughout the organization could be encouraged such as the sharing

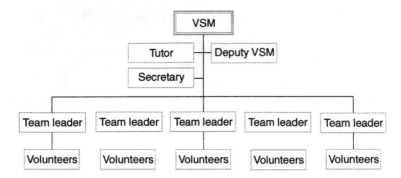

Figure 2.1 The management structure of a volunteer service.

of staff rooms, social events or a hospice internal newsletter to include both staff and volunteers.

Organizing the volunteer office

Good administrative back-up is a key to a successful volunteer service. Recruiting volunteers, keeping in touch with them, valuing their involvement with the organization can all be enhanced with efficient systems and record keeping. Providing skilled or trained volunteers in the right place at the right time is easier when accurate and up-to-date information is to hand. Planning for future projects or writing reports becomes more effective with the availability of statistics and data. Office accommodation is often in short supply, unless in purpose-built units, but as a minimum there should be sufficient space available to house the VSM and whatever staffing is agreed with access to at least one private room for interviewing volunteers.

Administrative support should be considered under the following headings:

1. Secretarial support, systems, and paperwork.

2. Record keeping.

3. Data collection.

Secretarial support, systems, and paperwork

Whatever resources are available, it is important to take time out to plan carefully what the needs of the department are, how best to deploy the office resources available and to design and develop efficient systems and procedures to help achieve the standards set down. Whether paperwork or computer systems are used it is vitally important that procedures are simple, clear, logical and consistent.

A high priority should be the appointment of a specific member of staff to oversee and co-ordinate the administrative systems in the volunteer office. There should be consistency of approach, a potential expert in word processing and computers, a supervisor for any extra volunteer administrative help. These will allow the VSM freedom from the minutiae of departmental organization. In reality, this is often not possible or sometimes only part-time hours are available. Whatever the circumstances, it is vital that the VSM does not attempt to undertake personally the administrative role. Much of the administrative support can, if there is no other alternative, be carried out by volunteers.

The VSM should not be afraid to delegate to volunteers such tasks as rota preparation, driving schedules, correspondence and liaison with other volunteers, meetings and training organization, and recruitment and selection administration. Since a number of different volunteers may have to be involved at any one time it is doubly important that the procedures in place are very clearly laid out and explained, that each volunteer knows exactly what is expected of them and who to report to in the case of any difficulties. Some volunteers will be happy to play a leading role, taking on more responsibility, perhaps in a supervisory capacity, while others will be happy to be directed to do some of the more straightforward tasks.[8]

If it is decided that volunteers are to be used to carry out the many administrative tasks, it is then important not to overlook the fact that attention must be paid to and sufficient resources allocated to accommodate a number of different people using equipment, such as telephones, computers, desks, chairs, etc.—perhaps at the same time as each other! Using volunteers is not necessarily a cheap option!

As computer technology develops and software packages become more available, investing in computer equipment should be another high priority. The requirements are likely to be complex and most volunteer departments will need a computer program with a wider capability than for a personnel department because of the range of information to be stored and processed. For example, the program may need to have the capacity to work out complicated volunteer rotas, taking into account constantly changing days and times of individual availability as well as holiday commitments. Currently in the UK, new software programs are being developed and coming on to the market, whilst some hospices, with the help of a resident expert (voluntary or staff), have developed their own packages. Whatever determines the decision taken, it is important that the organization has ready access to expertise to troubleshoot and develop the program to meet new requirements as these occur. Careful planning is key before committing to what might seem an expensive system. However, the benefits recouped in time and from the capability of a well-designed database, for example, will soon repay the outlay.

Record keeping

As in all personnel departments, a personal file should be kept on each individual volunteer. This should include such documents as the completed application form, references, interview documentation, and any subsequent paperwork in relation to the organization. Storage of these and access to them should be in line with local legislative and organizational guidelines (e.g. those on data protection).

Additional record-keeping systems will be developed according to the needs of the department. For example, the storing of detailed information on individual skills on offer from each volunteer, such as musical instruments played or languages spoken, may facilitate a speedy matching up of a request for help from the organization. Keeping records of attendance and starting dates provides readily available data when looking at long service or special awards. Tracking attendance and absence can flag potential problems for a volunteer. Acknowledging birthdays or an illness is a way of valuing volunteers. Recording training sessions attended and roles undertaken makes it easy to produce volunteer profiles.

Data collection

Report writing and forward planning are two elements of all managers' roles. Efficient data collection from volunteer records can provide such information as age distribution of volunteers, methods of recruitment, gender split, travelling costs, hours worked, training provided, etc. A well-designed data collection process can provide a large proportion of the fundamental information and statistics required. Further data on external factors will also be required and access to the World Wide Web via the Internet is an advantage.

The outreach factor

For a long time, the focus of the work of the VSM was with the volunteer work-force inside the hospice building. With the development of formal fund-raising activities in the community outside and, more recently, the advent of the retail arms of many hospices the involvement of volunteers has spread enormously. This has added to the pressure on the volunteer office as it is often expected that the VSM will add on the responsibility for these areas in many cases without extra resources. But the introduction of these 'different' volunteers also leads to other interesting questions such as how to make them feel part of the organization, how much training to offer, whether they should be treated in the same way as the hospice-based volunteers, etc. These questions amongst others should be discussed and agreed well in advance of developments. There is no rule that states that all volunteers have to come under the same remit of the volunteer office although it is important that there is consistency in the organization's approach to volunteers. In many hospices, the compromise is that the volunteer office has responsibility for volunteers who are required to complete an application form and become a registered volunteer (eg. those required to attend training sessions, team meetings, etc.).

Working to standards

Offering the highest possible quality of care to patients and their carers and families is the philosophy underpinning the work of all palliative care units. The contribution the volunteers and the volunteer service make should aim to enhance this quality of care wherever possible. To achieve this the volunteers must be willing to actively contribute to and support these standards of practice. This necessitates working to agreed guidelines and procedures within all departments. Establishing these with the departments concerned is the role of the VSM. Promoting the idea of working to standards should be apparent in all the volunteer documentation and communication with volunteers. A good example of this is the policy for 'confidentiality' which incorporates staff and volunteers alike.

Reviewing standards

The organization may already have a system of audit in place but, if not, this should not prevent the volunteer department from regularly reviewing its performance and looking at whether it can be improved. As long as aims, principal functions, policies and procedures are in place standards can be set.[3] Measuring what actually happens against the standards will produce information on how well targets are being met.

Continually reviewing in this way uncovers problems at an early stage, recognizes successes, promotes an open attitude to change and improvement, and can encourage participation and involvement in development from across the organization.

Conclusion

The role of the Voluntary Services Manager is thus a complex one encompassing many diverse responsibilities and requiring someone with a wide range of skills. The most important of these are the ability to communicate and motivate, followed very closely by good organizational skills. A capable and respected VSM can enable the organization to reap the benefit from a potential wealth of talent and time available in the community. A well-motivated and loyal volunteer workforce is a powerful link with that same community. Volunteers can be excellent ambassadors, educating the public about the work of the hospice and attracting new volunteers to support the hospice. The VSM is the vital link in that process.

References

1. Smith J D (1996). Should volunteers be managed? In (ed. David Billis and Margaret Harris), *Voluntary agencies, challenges of organization and management*, Ch. 12. Macmillan, London.
2. 'InVoLve'. *Quality programme for voluntary services departments in palliative care*. Help the Hospices, London.
3. Institute for Volunteering Research (IVR). (1997). *National survey of volunteering in the UK*. IVR, obtainable from 'InVoLve', c/o Help the Hospices, 34–44 Britannia St, London, WC1X 9JG.
4. Addington-Hall J and Karlson S (2001). *Summary of a national survey of health professionals and volunteers working in voluntary hospices*. Help the Hospices, London.
5. Field D and Johnson I (1993). Satisfaction and change: A survey of volunteers in a hospice organisation. Occasional Paper No. 8, April. Trent Palliative Care Centre (UK).

6. Scheier I H (1993). In *Building staff/volunteer relations*, Energize Books, Philadelphia, USA.
7. Hamilton G (1997). Volunteering: Team leadership. *Hospice Bulletin*, April, p. 1. The Hospice Information Service, St. Christopher's Hospice, London.
8. Plant H (1999). Working with volunteers—Team leaders. *Hospice Bulletin*, April, p. 7. The Hospice Information Service, St. Christopher's Hospice, London.

Recommended reading

Whitewood B (1999). The role of the volunteer in British palliative care. *European Journal of Palliative Care*, **6**(2).

Chapter 3

The position of the Volunteer Service Manager within the organization

It is the role of the Volunteer Service Manager (VSM) to recruit, develop, and motivate a large number of volunteers who make a substantial contribution to the economy and success of palliative care provision. The VSM provides this essential unpaid workforce to fit the changing needs of an organization and provides the right resources which enable senior managers to work with maximum efficiency. In order to succeed in this role it is crucially important that the VSM is placed at the right level in the organization's management structure. This chapter will explore this issue and the contribution of the VSM to overall management effectiveness and efficiency in the palliative care service.

The role of the VSM is different from other managers in the organization in that he/she has greater responsibility across the board to understand and provide creative staffing solutions in the different areas of activity in a hospice. The VSM can be viewed as the head of 'an organization within an organization', and can only carry out his/her role effectively if he/she has a place in the senior decision-making body of the palliative care provision.

This chapter aims to examine the role of the VSM in the context of the whole organization; its structure, mission, vision, and strategy. Principles of effective organizational structures will be demonstrated by describing roles and responsibilities at the first three tiers of strategic management, that of the Board, the Chief Executive, and the Senior Management Team. The chapter will explore a number of common structures in palliative care service management and examine them for their strengths and weaknesses. A number of recommendations will be made regarding the level at which the VSM should be placed within the structure of the organization according to the principles of good organizational design.

Deciding on an organizational structure

In order to achieve its goals any organization needs to have an *organizational structure*, a clearly defined hierarchy of authority. Ideally, staff need to have a good understanding of their own areas of responsibility and authority, as well as an equally clear comprehension of their own and all other roles within the organization.

An organizational structure provides a framework for, and more importantly determines, the nature of decision-making processes. Structure is also known to affect productivity, efficiency, organizational culture, and staff morale. Overlapping responsibilities and unclear reporting lines can be confusing. The resulting inefficiency may be exploited by individuals to the detriment of the organization.

The following questions can be a helpful checklist to guide decisions for people attempting to redesign or clarify the structure of an organization such as a hospice or palliative care service

◆ What kind of organization is it? What is its purpose?

◆ What does the organization aim to achieve now and in the future?

◆ What are the constraints on the organization? Internal, local, national, and legislative?

◆ At what stage is the organization in its life cycle? Is it newly formed or mature?

◆ What is the appropriate level in the organization for autonomous decision making?

◆ Should it be highly centralized at the top of the organization, or should responsibility for decisions and resources be placed at lower levels in the hierarchy?

◆ Who are the stakeholders who have a legitimate or informal interest in the organization? Patients, their families, Board of Trustees, senior managers, all paid and unpaid staff, donors, local community etc.?

◆ What basic positions should make up larger units?

◆ How should roles be grouped into departments and sections?

◆ What is the optimal number of staff reporting to one 'manager'? (The general recommendation is between 4 and 6 people reporting to one manager.)

These basic principles of effective organizational design apply to all organizations whether large, small voluntary or commercial.

The strategic planning process

Organizations determine their main purpose, future direction, and by what means they can fulfil and reach both, by the process of *strategic planning*. This should be an explicit process and is likely to be one of the main responsibilities of the Board and the Chief Executive. Depending on the predictability of future circumstances a decision needs to be made on the appropriate number of years of each planning cycle. Twenty years ago most strategic plans used to span between three and five years, but in the recent climate of increasingly rapid and unpredictable change, planning cycles have shortened to two to three years. This strategic planning process is best carried out with the help of a facilitator,

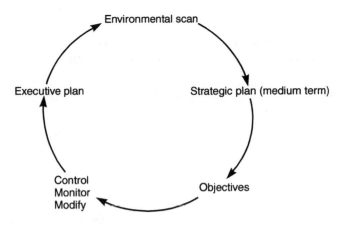

Figure 3.1 The strategic planning cycle.

preferably from outside the organization, who takes the planning group away from the company and guides them through the process of strategy formulation. Figure 3.1 demonstrates the sequence of the strategic planning process.

Mission

All organizations need to determine their main purpose, future direction and by what means these can be reached. *Organizational mission* is the reason or purpose for which it exists. It is a broad statement of philosophy and values, with an emotional content that represents the basic spirit of the organization and takes into account the perspective of the customer or service receiver. Mission statements need to be short, value-based rather than specific, and must endure over time.

An example of a mission statement.

- We believe that our patients, their families and friends are the centre of everything we do.
- We believe we should meet the individual needs of people with life-threatening illnesses, and those who care for them with dignity. These needs may be physical, emotional or psychological.
- We believe we should provide a unique and specialized service complementary to, and in partnership with the local health care provisions.
- We recognize that the commitment to quality assurance by everyone in the organization is vital to our mission.
- We recognize that we need to manage our resources in a caring, efficient, and cost-effective manner.
- We believe we should provide an environment in which feelings may be expressed and acknowledged with sensitivity.

Vision

The *vision* of an organization's future will not only set a context in which actions will be taken, but also help to point it in a certain direction.

An example of a vision for the future.

The Hospice will aim to raise sufficient funds to build a children's unit in the next five years, while maintaining the high level of palliative care for existing patients.

Both the mission and the vision are motivators to work towards shared goals and values. It is these aspects that can provide psychological commitment to the organization from staff, those they are there to serve and other stakeholders. *Such commitment can only be achieved if the mission and vision are explicitly communicated to all staff, and demonstrated by both the words and actions of the Board, Chief Executive, and the Senior Management Team.*

The strategic plan

The *strategic plan* is the means by which an organization can reach its goals. Strategy builds on the mission and vision as a context within which it defines its goals. Strategic plans tend to span a period of between two to five years depending on the type and speed of change in the environment. The strategic plan is the catalyst that turns intentions into activity.

There are usually five phases in the determination of strategy:

1 analysis.

2 options.

3 formulation of the plan and objectives.

4 communication and implementation.

5 evaluation of achievements.

Analysis allows for the scanning of both internal and external environments. It highlights opportunities, threats, strengths, and weaknesses and is likely to clarify a number of strategic options. When choosing an option it is good practice to use strengths and opportunities to combat perceived threats and weaknesses.

At the implementation phase, the strategy needs to be widely communicated and explained to all staff. This can be done either on a cascading basis, with managers briefing their own staff, or as an organizational event, where the Chief Executive makes a presentation to all staff. It is important at this stage that the strategic plan is translated into objectives. Staff at all levels needs to ask themselves the question: 'if this is the strategy, what does it mean for us in this department?'

A well-formulated strategy gives clear guiding principles for setting appropriate objectives. Objectives need to state in *precise measurable* terms with time limits what is to be achieved and who has the main responsibility for an objective. An example of a *badly* phrased objective might be: '*To improve the quality of patient care*'. This objective does not answer the question of how will we know when and how quality of patient care has improved?

The following objectives set by a VSM are more appropriate:

The VSM to design and implement an integrated volunteer appraisal system by 30 November 2003. The appraisal system will be:

- linked to appropriate training, relevant to the needs of the hospice;
- communicated to and understood by volunteers and staff;
- simple to administer;
- linked to individual development of volunteers.

Methods of control and monitoring need to be built into the strategic plan at the time of its formulation. The plan needs to allow for flexibility so that it can be modified in the light of changes in the internal or external environment. It is one of the principal responsibilities of the Board to monitor the implementation and progress of the strategic plan.

At the end of each planning period it is useful to look back on achievements and difficulties in order to incorporate such learning into the formulation of the plans for the next phase.

Organizational structure

There are a number of basic types of organizational structures that can be used to implement strategy. Figure 3.2 shows the senior levels of a typical functional organizational structure often adopted by middle sized companies. Starting at the top of the organization, the Board, with its Chairman, constitutes the Corporate Governance of the organization.

The major roles of the Board are to:

- define corporate mission and vision;
- determine the fundamental principles and policies of the organization;
- judge strategic initiatives against environmental changes;

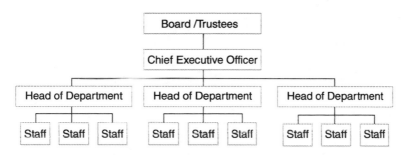

Figure 3.2 The functional organizational structure.

- select and manage the Chief Executive;
- ensure that the planning process fits with the mission;
- monitor overall performance of the organization;
- network on behalf of the organization and communicate with major stakeholders;
- take ultimate responsibility for the organization meeting its legal duties.

Board members each have specific responsibility for areas of the organization's strategy reflecting their knowledge and expertise. The various committees of the Board need to have a defined and agreed remit and terms of reference to aim for.

An example of the terms of reference for a Clinical Governance and Quality Committee of a Board of Trustees in a UK Hospice

Terms of reference

- Set clear standards of service care, following guidance of the National Institute of Clinical Effectiveness, and National Council for Hospice and Specialist Palliative Care Services.
- Audit and evaluate care.
- Monitor changes in practice as a result of audit.
- Encourage innovative research to improve patient care.
- Ensure best use of resources in the achievement of high standards.
- Encourage culture where staff and their work is valued.
- Ensure development of relevant competence and expertise of all clinical staff to meet standards set.

Membership

Chief Executive
Two Trustees
Medical Director
Palliative Care Consultant
Patient Services Manager
Volunteer Services Manager
Education Manager
Consumer Representative

(Continued)

Terms of office

Members will be reviewed every three years.

Frequency of meeting

Three times per year.

Reporting to

Chairman of Trustees.

The *Chairman* (or Chairperson in modern parlance) of the Board is a figurehead who represents the organization on important public occasions. The Chairman is responsible for the performance of the Board and the line management of the Chief Executive.

The Chairman of the Board and its members are often senior managers in other organizations, which do not compete or conflict with their membership of the Board in question. They are not employees of the company, but bring a specific expertise or status, and receive only token payments and expenses in return for their work. This gives them the relative independence needed for this strategic role. In a sense they are volunteers (see Chapters 4 and 5). Boards tend to meet quarterly, or monthly in rapidly changing situations.

The *Chief Executive* is the most senior staff member, responsible for the organization's strategic objectives and allocating appropriate resources to meet these objectives as well as being responsible for the implementation of decisions, principles, and policies determined by the Board. One of the most challenging aspects of the Chief Executive's role is to successfully manage communication with the Chair and members of the Board.

The Chief Executive is the line manager of the members of the Senior Management Team and usually chairs its meetings

The Senior Management Team (SMT)

All members of the SMT have their own assigned responsibility and final authority for an area of operation within the organization. Depending on the level of centralization they also have their own budgets and are able to make decisions on resource allocations. In addition to their specific areas of expertise and authority, members of the SMT act as a strategic forum under the chairmanship of the Chief Executive. For these cross boundary strategic activities they have to make decisions about what is best for the organization, even if it is not particularly advantageous to their areas of operation. In this forum they represent the organization as a whole. This dual responsibility may not sit easily

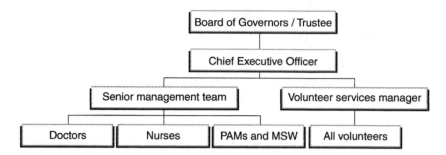

Figure 3.3 Management structure: Model A.

with all members of the SMT. Specialized training in strategic planning ought to be a prerequisite for membership at this level of the organization.

The position of the VSM in the organizational structure

According to a recent unpublished survey of all UK hospices and palliative care services, only 23% of Volunteer Service Managers (VSMs) are members of the Senior Management Team, where they can make a direct input into hospice strategy and policy in their own right. This statistic shows how underrated and underutilized the majority of VSMs in the UK are at this stage of the development of hospice and palliative care. The same survey also showed that in most hospices the post has evolved into a paid one from that of a voluntary one, often with little evaluation or planning. However, there are still 6% of VSMs who are unpaid volunteers.

It is the responsibility of the Trustees and the Chief Executive to place this post at the appropriate level within the hospice's structure, and acknowledge the scope and importance of this role.

The following models of management structures illustrate how the differing perceptions of the role of the VSM are reflected in their place in the organization's structure.

Model A (Figure 3.3) illustrates a structure where the VSM reports to the Chief Executive, and is on the same level as, but not part of, the Senior Management Team. While this model acknowledges the importance of the role it may leave the VSM separated from other senior managers and does not allow for adequate participation in the strategic decision-making body of the hospice. The volunteers and their manager appear as an isolated unit rather than as valued participants in the functioning of the hospice.

The structure implies that all volunteers are managed by the VSM and do not report to managers in the departments of the hospice where they may carry out their duties. This would not only be a cause of frustration and misunderstanding, but would also leave the VSM with an impossibly large span of control.

Model B (Figure 3.4) places the VSM as a member of the Senior Management Team, where the post-holder can be party to decisions and planning with his/her colleagues. This is probably the most appropriate positioning of the role at the

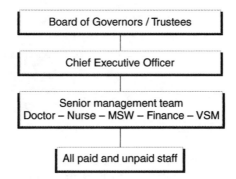

Figure 3.4 Management structure: Model B.

present level of hospice development and representative of the positions held by the 23% of the VSMs in the UK.

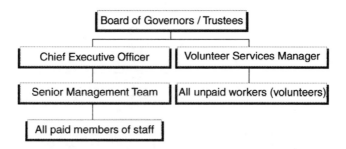

Figure 3.5 Management structure: Model C.

Model C (Figure 3.5) places the VSM at the same level in the structure as that of the Chief Executive, and, like the latter, reporting to the Board of Trustees. This structure once again separates the VSM role from the Senior Management Team.

It views paid and unpaid staff as autonomous groups within the organization. This model represents a structure that does not enhance the level of integration necessary for most hospices to achieve their strategic goals. Most hospices are small or medium sized organizations with less than a hundred employees. This model suggests that there are two equally important and responsible posts at the top of a relatively small organization. This kind of structure is liable to generate conflict between the two halves, and the construction of unproductive alliances.

Model D (Figure 3.6) is representative of a large percentage of hospices surveyed, where the VSM reports to a senior manager and is placed on the third tier of the organization. There is no Chief Executive or Senior Management Team. They are replaced by the heads of what are regarded as the three major groups within the hospice, that of medicine, nursing, and administration.

This structure has a number of disadvantages. There is no uniting role between the three functions except for the Board of Trustees, who are not full-time and are not employees of the organization. The managers heading the three functions

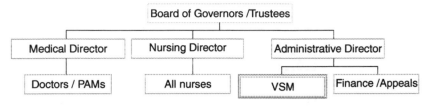

Figure 3.6 Management structure: Model D.

would therefore not each have the support of a line manager. The VSM is seen as part of the administrative function with little or no influence or input at the appropriate level. This type of structure does not reflect the challenges of the present environment in the hospice movement.

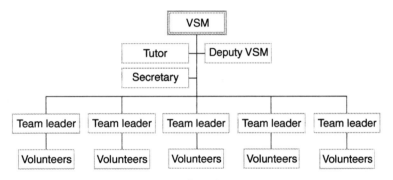

Figure 3.7 The management structure of a volunteer structure.

The management structure of the volunteer service

Important as it is that the Volunteer Service Manager is appropriately placed within the management structure to reflect the importance of the volunteer service and his/her contribution to the management of the unit, it has to be remembered that there also has to be a structure within the volunteer service itself. This is illustrated in Figure 3.7, already mentioned in Chapter 2.

The VSM is at the head, carrying ultimate responsibility for the service, its workers and everything to do with them (selection, training, support, supervision, etc.). He/she is assisted by others each responsible for an aspect of volunteer work—flower arranging, coffee shops, sitting with patients, transport service, charity shops, etc. They are often termed 'team leaders'. If their team is particularly large they too may have assistants or deputies. Many volunteer services have someone solely concerned with the pre-service and ongoing training of volunteers, answerable directly to the VSM. The team leaders, trainers and the VSM meet, as a management team, at regular but not necessarily frequent intervals under the chairmanship of the VSM. In effect, they form the Senior Management Team of the volunteer service.

Moving into the future

These organizational models illustrate a number of structures that make different assumptions of the importance and contribution of the Volunteer Service Manager. The processes of strategic planning and development of organizational structure, mentioned earlier in this chapter are tools only recently used by the more forward-looking Boards and Chief Executives. The present and future environment within which hospices need to survive and succeed will be helped by the strong set of values that drive them. However, these values will not be sufficient to meet the demands to be faced. In order to increase the chances of success, hospices and palliative care services need to embrace a more strategic approach to planning and organizational structure. The structure of an organization will serve its purpose best when it is appropriate for tackling the challenges of the environment and the strategic objective.

The contribution of the volunteer workforce lends flexibility and a rich resource base to the hospice. In order to best utilize this resource the role and professionalism of the VSM needs to be recognized by placing him/her at the Senior Management Team level of the organization, and ensuring that the volunteer service is well integrated into this policy and decision-making body of the hospice. At present in the UK, over 60% of VSMs have a degree or professional qualification, and the majority recognize the need to make their role a professional one in the near future. The challenge is clear both for the VSMs and those who manage them.

Chapter 4

The selection of volunteers

Why do we need a process of selection?

Palliative care and specialist palliative care provision involves working at the 'sharp end' of health care, with people made vulnerable through illness and an unrelenting prognosis. This care may be provided through a charity, private or government-funded health care provisions all of which may 'employ' volunteers to enhance/complement their service. Regardless of funding the patients, their carers and families have expectations of palliative care services to provide quality care and support, safely and competently adhering to national and international standards.

In the selection of volunteers we are:

- exercising a legal and moral obligation, a duty of care;
- choosing the best and most appropriate people for our organization;
- not just choosing the right people but choosing the right people at the right time for both the organization and the individual;
- identifying potential, looking for those who have the capacity for development and growth—who will blossom in and enhance the palliative care environment;
- protecting to the best of our ability those people in the organization's care—patients, carers, paid staff and volunteers—from physical, emotional, and spiritual harm.

Poor selection of voluntary staff can lead to disruption, conflict, and harm to individuals and the organization.

According to Smith[1] an organization can adopt one of three selection approaches but these can often overlap:

1 *Non-rejection*—nobody is rejected because there is always some job suitable.

2 *Recruitment*—recruited and selected for a specific task only—similar to paid employment techniques.

3 *Matching*—looking at what the volunteer is presenting and finding a job to match.

The selection of volunteers can fit into three main groups:

1 **Recruited** (active recruitment by the hospice):
   - blanket recruitment (a general appeal for volunteers);
   - recruitment for a specific area of work, for example, day care or for a specific task (e.g. as a driver).

2 **Unsolicited applications:** Individuals or groups independent of recruitment drives approach the organization with a wish to volunteer, with or without a specific task in mind.

3 **Work experience**/student training placements/government schemes: These can be at the individual's request or a condition of qualifying either for training/employment or for government benefits, e.g. unemployment benefits.

The selection process

Selection is a dynamic process—it has specific criteria that must be met along the way but it also enables some flexibility to accommodate individual circumstances and professional judgement. The selection process consists of the following components the order of which will vary with organizational policy and personal preference:

- Application
- References
- Interview
- Induction
- Probation

Throughout the process of selection the Volunteer Service Manager (VSM) uses a combination of:

- Interpersonal and communication skills
- Experience
- Professional judgement
- Discretion
- Intuition
- Gut feeling

Judgement is needed to determine the weight of each factor as it is presented. Written, verbal, and non-verbal communications are examined in order to make a value judgement whilst ensuring that he/she and other members of staff are not being manipulated.

Some of the skills needed by a VSM when selecting volunteers.

- Informal and formal interview technique and skills—interpretation of verbal and non-verbal messages.
- Using open and closed questions.
- Basic counselling/communication skills—listening, empathy, paraphrasing or rephrasing, summarizing, giving feedback.
- Breaking bad news—handling and understanding rejection.

There are five stages in the selection process, which are clearly illustrated in Figures 4.1 and 4.2. *The crucially important difference between the two is when confidential reports ('references') are called for and used.* Some interviewers prefer to have seen them and have them in front of them when they see the applicant. Others only call for them after the interview. There are points in favour of each.

It should be noted that the selection process permits rejection as well as selection. Rejection, for whatever reason, may take place at various stages of the process, as illustrated in Figures 4.1 and 4.2 and discussed below

The basis for selection

The Voluntary Service Manager and management colleagues must decide on what will they judge the suitability of an applicant. Will it be primarily on the:

- Application form?
- Past history?
- References?
- Interview—information ascertained and gut feeling?

Application

Application will involve the completion of an application form either written or submitted on the Internet on a secure site to maintain confidentiality. A designated person must be made responsible for applications coming in, for acknowledging them and for calling for references, to ensure confidentiality and best practice.

The application form differs from the forms used to employ paid staff but should observe a similar equal opportunity, non-discriminatory, confidential approach. In general, the emphasis will be on life experience, skills, and motivation rather than on qualifications. However, when recruiting for a specific task or an application to work in a 'qualified' capacity (e.g. complementary therapies), then specific qualifications will be required that meet with an agreed/approved

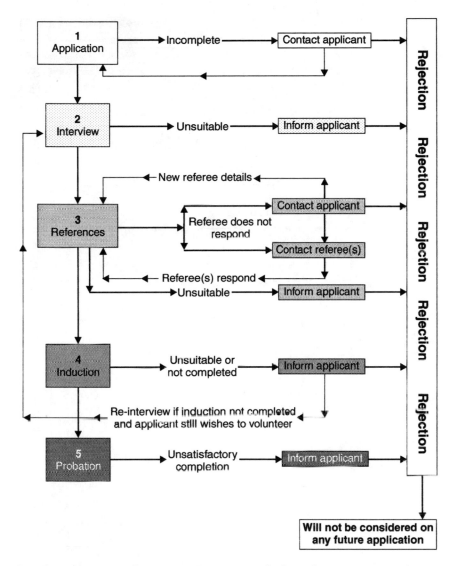

Figure 4.1 Five-stage selection criteria. Interview *before* references requested (from: S A Spencer Grey 2001).

competency pathway (i.e. a minimum requirement of professional bodies and/or the organization).

An equal opportunities statement must be included on the form—non-discriminatory with regard to gender, sexual orientation, creed, colour, religion, level of ability or disability.

Carefully thought-out 'open' questions should be used where possible, with strategically placed closed questions to prevent ambiguity in crucial areas (e.g. criminal convictions). The questions should be kept to a minimum.

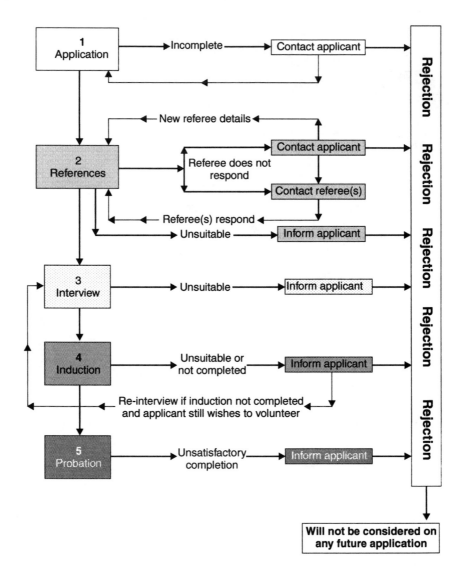

Figure 4.2 Five-stage selection criteria. Interview with references *already* provided (from S A Spencer Grey 2001).

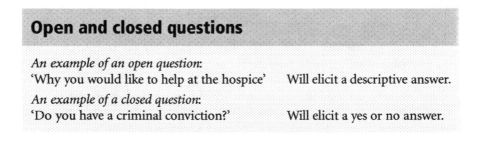

Open and closed questions

An example of an open question:
'Why you would like to help at the hospice'   Will elicit a descriptive answer.

An example of a closed question:
'Do you have a criminal conviction?'   Will elicit a yes or no answer.

What is the *minimum* information you need to get from this form?

- Name.
- Address.
- Health status.
- Criminal convictions.
- Motivation.
- What they would like to do to help.
- Names and addresses of two referees.

What is the *minimum* information you will give in this form?

- Organizational details—name, address etc., registered charity number.
- Name and job title of contact person.
- Confidentiality explanation—regarding details given by the applicant and regarding the nature of hospice work. (Some organizations include a confidentiality statement to be signed and returned with the application form. It would be better practice to sign this statement at a later stage after the meaning and implications of confidentiality have been carefully discussed with the volunteer, see Chapter 13.)
- Mention should be made of the particular stresses that can be encountered in hospice work and palliative care—alluding to recent bereavement, etc. (This can be done either on the application form or in an accompanying leaflet that gives details of volunteer opportunities available, etc.)
- A brief explanation as to who to give as a referee.
- The need for honesty and openness (e.g. declaring criminal convictions).

The language used in these forms will be less formal than normally used in application forms with explanations accompanying terminology to ensure they are easy to understand, feel non-threatening, and encourage openness and honesty. It may be worth having the application form and explanatory notes checked for 'Plain English'[2] to ensure that the language used has been kept simple and straightforward.

Those people with poor literacy skills or sensory disablement may need assistance with the completion of their application forms. This can be facilitated by:

- Applicant being accompanied/assisted by a witness/advocate.
- Audio or videotape recordings of application interviews.

In the case of an incomplete or unsatisfactory completion of the application form

Contact applicant—by letter or telephone, providing a contact name and number:

- either requesting more information or the name of another referee; *or*
- informing the applicant they have been unsuccessful at this time.

Such phone calls can be difficult. Document them in the applicant's notes or in their computer entry. If it is considered a difficult call (having decided that it really is necessary in the first place) then it may be recorded *with the applicant having been informed*, or conducted in the hearing of others, *again with the applicant having been informed*. Permission or consent for witnesses or recording from the applicant is not necessary but they must be informed of any action you are taking.

Key issue: This is the first point in the selection process when an applicant may be rejected.

References/confidential reports

Usually two references or 'confidential reports' will be required. The purpose of these references and the assurance of confidentiality must be made clear to the applicant.

If possible, one of these referees should be their current or last employer but otherwise they can be friends or colleagues but they *cannot* be relatives. Some organizations may call for a doctor's reference and some may tailor their references to the job involved.

It is the responsibility of the prospective employer, not the applicant, to call for these reports from the people named by the applicant.

Key issue: Do you request references before or after interview? What are the 'pros' and 'cons'?

Calling for confidential reports

- Use a standard letter requesting reports and enclose a standard form.
- Enclose a 'prepaid' addressed envelope (makes it easier to return).
- Listen to verbal/telephone references (they may prefer to speak to someone rather than fill in forms).
- Act on verbal leads where appropriate.
- Do not accept letters of recommendation presented by the applicant without further verification—these are not what is meant by confidential reports or references.

Key issue: Do you inform the applicant that rejection was because of a confidential report? How much information do you give about it? Will it embarrass the person providing the report? Should you inform the referee of the rejection?

Interview

The interview suggested here takes place *before* induction but it is appreciated that this will not be every organization's policy. Other options include:

(1) interview after induction; and

(2) interviews before and after induction.

The interview is often called an 'informal interview', 'a meeting' or 'a visit' to make it feel less threatening. There are two ways of identifying suitability for interview (see Figures 4.1 and 4.2).

(1) from information provided on the application form; and

(2) from such information *plus* information from confidential reports.

The approach adopted will depend on personal preference and organizational policy. In either option, the interview may have been conducted at the same time as completion of the application form if assistance with this was required. Progression to induction will still depend on receipt of suitable references.

> **Key issue**: What part will police checks play in your selection process, when will they be selected and how will the information be used?

Selection by interview *before* induction can prevent waste of time and money for both the organization and the applicant. It may also prevent feelings of resentment in unsuccessful applicants who felt that going through an induction was equated with acceptance. This in turn helps to preserve the good name of the organization and demonstrates good practice.

It is worth remembering that people volunteer for a reason and that reason needs to be ascertained. Putting applicants at ease helps the VSM to discover that reason. *The interview itself should be as informal as possible.* It should:

* put people at their ease;
* encourage spontaneous divulging of information—often of a personal nature;
* allow applicants to express their personality;
* allow for expression of feelings—about themselves, others, and situations;
* allow for expression of beliefs—religious and non-religious, values—what they hold dear and attitudes—their opinions, their way of thinking and behaving;
* enable investigation and discussion of motivation. Why are they here, what do they want from the experience, what do they feel they can contribute?

Considerations when conducting an informal interview are:

* preparation.
* the venue.
* who is going to be present/conduct the interview?

- interview structure.
- equity.

Some of these issues are discussed by Steve McCurley and Rick Lynch in their book.[3]

Preparation

- Arrange interview times with space between interviews to allow for delays and some thinking time.
- Book and prepare the venue—availability, comfortable chairs, refreshments, etc.
- Have the volunteer's information present—application form, references—read these before the interview.
- Have a list of the jobs available with descriptions and required criteria.
- Have your questions prepared—there will be general questions and job/task specific ones—are you going to use an interview record form?
- Have information available to give to the potential volunteers about their chosen area of work, the organization, and confidentiality—*should they sign a confidentiality statement at this time?*

The venue

The interview may be conducted in an office, a designated interview or counselling room or designed to ensure:

- privacy;
- comfort; and
- uninterrupted 'quality time'.

If the volunteer feels they are in the way, being rushed or they are being interviewed in an open or shared office they will not feel valued. If they are made to feel unimportant they are less likely to 'open up' and will not form a favourable opinion of the person conducting the interview or ultimately of the organization. First impressions last!

Who is going to be present/conduct the interview?

The interview is usually conducted as a 'one-to-one'. On the whole, this is less intimidating. However, if you are interviewing for a specific post or role it might be advantageous to collaborate with the line manager/supervisor there as well. This will ensure that all the needs of the post are being met, the staff are happy with the allocation, and it also improves interdepartmental relationships.

The interviewer will normally be the VSM or a person designated by him/her to conduct interviews in his/her absence. The interviewer must have some informal interview knowledge and skills training.

The safety of the VSM/interviewer must be considered at all times. As a safety precaution and to ensure privacy, other staff must be made aware that an interview is taking place as well as where, when and who is conducting it. If the interviewer feels uncomfortable about an interview for some reason—this could be a gender issue or because of the likelihood of rejection—then another staff member may be invited to attend the interview. The interviewee must be informed that a third person will be present but this can be done subtly so that they do not feel this is an unusual occurrence.

Interview structure

An interview has a beginning, a middle and an end.

The *beginning* or opening—build a rapport and put them at their ease.

- Make the volunteer feel welcome, and thank him/her for showing an interest in the organization and taking the time to attend.

- Explain the purpose of the interview—to find out more about each other (organization and volunteer), to identify any suitable positions for that individual and to come to a decision (mutual) as to the suitability of volunteering with this organization. Ensure the volunteer knows he/she is free to ask questions at any time during the interview process.

Selection is a two-way process that belongs as much to the volunteer as to the organization. The volunteer can reject the organization. If it is considered that the applicant is unsuitable you can subtly and constructively steer the opinions and discussion so that it is the volunteer that chooses not to continue with the application.

The *middle*—information exchange and assessment/appraisal of the volunteer.

- Here, detailed information about the work of the hospice is given to include confidentiality, the sensitive nature of this work and some of the particular stress or consequences of this (e.g. bereavement). Available jobs are discussed to include their importance to the organization and to the patients, identifying the skills and/or qualifications needed for each.

- Most of the interview is going to be about getting the volunteers to talk about themselves, their interests, their skills, and their motivation. Give volunteers time to discuss the available jobs. How would they approach the work? What training do they feel they need? This can give some insight into attitudes to the hospice/work/patients involved and also shows how they perceive themselves and their needs.

Looking out for different personality traits/elements can help you identify a job match for a volunteer and can also help to assess suitability for volunteering. There are many different areas to look out for whilst interviewing. For example:

- Ease in answering questions about personal attributes and background—are they trying to hide something, are they embarrassed by a lack of qualifications?

- Ability to communicate well—do they use inappropriate language, do they have difficulty in expressing themselves?

- Level of enthusiasm and commitment. General attitudes and emotional reactions—do they show overwhelming emotion or prejudices?

- Types of questions they ask about the organization and the position on offer—does this seem a healthy interest?

- Other interests and hobbies—life should be about balance. If the individual does not seem to have any other interests in life and they want to commit most of their time to the organization it has to be questioned is this healthy for them and the organization?
- Flexibility and reliability. Maturity and stability—this is not always associated with age.
- Do they want to work as part of a team—does this have implications for team working, for supervision, and for taking instruction?
- Level of self-confidence—do they seem lacking in confidence or do they seem over-confident and 'know it all'? Any sense of a hidden agenda—can you tackle them about this?
- Patterns in previous jobs and volunteering—do they show poor attendance or unreliability? Reasons for coming to the interview—genuine wish to volunteer, because they were told to in order to claim benefits etc., just to see what the hospice was about? To gain some interview experience?
- Preferences in type of work—a volunteer can be adamant about patient contact or bereavement counselling when this is clearly unsuitable given their references, skills and personal history—this shows poor self-awareness or may indicate a hidden agenda? A volunteer wanting no patient contact at all (e.g. wanting to work in one of the charity shops) can be better understood perhaps.

Although each interview will be tailored to the individual the same areas of discussion and information will be included each time. The use of an interview form will help maintain quality, consistency and equity.

The *end*

At the end of the interview what are you offering?—a position? induction? training (e.g. as a bereavement support worker?). Give clear details of the next stage of the process with time scales and expectations.

In the case of training as a bereavement support worker, home care visitor, etc., it must be made clear that a further selection interview is necessary after successful completion of their training. The training will not automatically guarantee that individual a position in that area of work.

Equity

To 'treat everybody the same' does not provide equity. Equity in this instance means that regardless of socio-economic status, race, gender, sexual orientation, ethnicity, culture, and/or disability an individual will have equal opportunity to access information about, be able to apply to be and have equal chance of selection as a volunteer. Equity actions are deliberate efforts to ensure that services and information are flexible in form and function to ensure equal access to all—they eliminate bias, streotyping, and discrimination. Access for all will permeate all aspects of the hospice and palliative care provision and will adhere to statutory obligations (Acts of Law) and to your organization's equal opportunities policy and code of conduct. Selection criteria for all posts must be clearly defined and reflected in the information sent to applicants, which must also include details of the organization's commitment to equality of opportunity.

> The interview is the second point in the selection process when an applicant may be rejected.

Applicant is found unsuitable at interview

There may be several reasons for rejection at this stage:

1 *Unsuitable as a volunteer:*
  - inform applicant there and then
  - give reasons for not being selected—use discretion and ensure own safety. (*Safety will include potential violence, sexual harassment, physical harm or verbal abuse but also includes protection from false accusations.*)
  - thank them once again for the interest they have shown and for the time they have given

2 *Unsuitable for their chosen area of work:*
  - give reasons for not being selected—use discretion and ensure own safety;
  - if appropriate, offer a review meeting in 6 months time (e.g. the applicant has had a recent bereavement). It is a good idea to set a time for a review, as this will be interpreted as positive rather than as just 'a brush off';
  - thank them once again for the interest they have shown and for the time they have given.

3 *No vacancies in the requested area:*
  - offer another work area or put on a waiting list for their chosen area—these offers may or may not be accepted; thank them once again for the interest they have shown and for the time they have given.

Before potential volunteers leave after the informal interview ensure:
  - any paperwork or permission has been completed/sought (confidentiality statement, references); they have an opportunity to ask questions;
  - they have clear information to take away:
    - contact details,
    - time and date of the next appointment,
    - details of the further 'selection hoops' and points of rejection.

A successful interview will result in the applicant processing to the next stage of the selection process.

Induction

The details of an induction programme are discussed in Chapter 5. Here, induction is mentioned because it is a part of the selection process and needs to be completed successfully to enable further progression towards final selection. Induction can be a day, half a day or series of sessions (e.g. weekly). All volunteers must attend induction. It will incorporate the basic legal requirements for insurance, health and safety, and confidentiality. Departmental induction in this chapter is referred to as part of probation.

Induction is the third point where an applicant may be rejected.

Unsuitability of an applicant or non-attendance

1 A person may interview well but during induction as part of a group or team they may show poor interaction, communication, and team skills or may be very domineering, which may—depending on the role to be fulfilled—show the applicant to be unsuitable.

2 They may fail to attend some or the entire induction programme.

The VSM should then:

• Contact the applicant—in writing, in person or by phone.

• Set up an informal interview, if appropriate to:

  – discuss/consider mitigating circumstances,

  – discuss attitude/behaviour—use discretion and ensure own safety,

  – put further selection processes in place (e.g. review date).

• Reject by letter or by telephone.

If a volunteer has not completed the mandatory parts of their induction (e.g. health and safety, moving and handling, fire, confidentiality, etc.) in the timescales dictated by the organization they cannot commence or continue work.

The protocol for induction will vary among organizations (e.g. volunteers can attend their place of work four times before induction or they must receive induction within six weeks of commencing work, etc.).

If the volunteer having been given every opportunity to attend the required session(s) does not complete but still wishes to volunteer then they will have to be re-interviewed and a risk assessment conducted as to their likelihood of attendance and completion of the mandatory requirements. Time and resources must be considered, as must the commitment and motivation of the individual. It could be a waste of time and money for both applicant and the Volunteer Service Manager.

Probation

The purpose of a probation period is to give the new volunteer and the organization time to see if they have made the right choice. It is the time to set up suitable means of support and supervision and enables necessary training and assessment of skills and competency. It is a 'getting to know you' period.

This period is most often supervised by the managers/designated supervisors/team leaders in that work area rather than directly by the VSM. A planned departmental induction and competency criteria is agreed between the manager and volunteer. The criteria and induction package should have previously been agreed with the VSM adhering to the organization's induction strategy and established competency pathways.

During the probation period there may be some mandatory training to be undertaken (e.g. the use of hoists), but this time is also about being shown the 'ropes', being supervised, advised, and supported by a designated staff member (trained in mentorship/supervision) until the new volunteer applicant feels confident and competent and the mentor/team leader endorses this according to agreed criteria.

Throughout the probation period the VSM is informed of the volunteer's progress by the line manager/team leader who will conduct regular reviews (formal or informal) with the volunteer. Any problems that the volunteer or staff experience should be discussed with the VSM including any interpersonal or work conflicts, and a strategy for handling the situation to be decided between the VSM, the volunteer and supervisory staff involved—protocols should be established for this. Sometimes, the practicalities of volunteers meeting with their mentors/supervisors can be difficult because of shifts, holidays, etc., and so their competency is not being properly assessed in agreed timescales or by the designated supervisors. If this situation persists then the system used must be examined to see if it can be improved.

If the volunteer does not meet the probationary requirements by the end of the probation period an extension can be granted in some circumstances if the staff in that area and the VSM agree that is the best way forward. If the volunteer is considered to be unsuitable or he/she is unhappy in that particular volunteer role he/she may be offered an alternative work area or they may be asked to leave.

An interview at the end of a successful probation period is a good idea. This is usually conducted by the VSM or the team leader in that area of volunteer work it marks the end of their probationary period, tells the volunteer what they have done well, where they can improve, but mainly it is a recognition of their commitment and welcomes them aboard.

Dismissal or removal, at any time, of a volunteer from a work area should be authorized by the VSM after consultation with the staff and with the volunteer concerned—protocols should be established for this.

Probation is the fourth point in the selection process where an applicant may be rejected.

Rejecting an applicant during / on completion of the probation period

◆ Inform the probationer—in person, at a planned interview and in writing.
◆ Give reasons for not being selected—use discretion and ensure own safety.

Rejection of an applicant at any stage in the process

The VSM should handle rejection firmly, fairly and sensitively—think about how it feels to be rejected. When handling rejection:

◆ Temper with positive feedback.

◆ Suggest alternatives or ways forward.

◆ Highlight the positives of that individual.

◆ Maybe direct them towards another more suitable agency or towards some training that may be of benefit to them and to future applications.

◆ Try not to lie or couch the truth too heavily.

◆ Be constructive especially regarding criticism.

Bending the rules

From experience, a situation that the VSM and other staff may be confronted with is when a colleague, a manager or a volunteer encourages the moving of a volunteer to another work area or brings in a new volunteer *without going through the normal volunteer selection system*.

This is unsafe practice and should be dealt with quickly and effectively but sensitively as well as firmly. Often, the individuals involved do not see the significance of their actions and can be quite shocked and upset by the reaction that their 'just trying to help' can cause.

> **Key issue:** If a selection policy and process are to be successful, the VSM must be a member of the senior management team and have their professional respect and support at all times. Breaches in the process usually point to the need for improved management and a review of policies.

Implementing the selection process

The selection standards and policies must be clear, robust, realistic—a true representation of the system in place—whilst reflecting the palliative care unit's philosophy of care, protection, and integrity. The documents defining selection and the policy underpinning it must be circulated and made freely available to all managers and staff, paid and unpaid. Education in the importance of the volunteer selection process may be included in the induction programme.

Selection of Trustees

In a charitable organization, such as many hospices and palliative care services, the most senior management is most often the Board of Trustees who carry ultimate legal responsibility for the running of the unit.

This section has been included here because, although the VSM may not be involved in Trustee selection, he/she they may well be involved in their induction.

Some Trustees will also work as volunteer staff within the hospice and an understanding of some of the issues around Trustees may be useful to highlight potential conflicts of interest and management problems.

The Trustees are often the founding volunteers who helped to create the organizations and defined its aims and objectives, decided the structure, policy, and philosophy, and often hold a legal and financial responsibility within the organization. As a result, they may have a strong feeling of ownership.[4] Within the framework they created they made space for others like themselves—volunteers—partly in recognition of their monetary value and partly to allow others to gain the same sense of worth and achievement and satisfaction that they have experienced.[3–5]

As an organization develops the Trustees will change as will the qualities and they skills they bring to the work. As time passes, fewer and fewer Trustees are the founding volunteers and more specific skills-based selection and recruitment may take place. The role of the Trustee changes as an organization grows and the role and responsibilities of Trustees must be clearly defined to ensure effective management and achievement of goals.[4,5]

The eligibility criteria for Trustees will vary but will reflect that organization's constitution and 'company' and legal status. But there are some common features of a Board of Trustees:

- Most Trustees are selected from the organization's 'members' or 'friends' or its volunteer workforce.
- There may be 'time-served' criteria in place (e.g. five years as a volunteer, etc.).
- A Trustee position is usually a voluntary (i.e. unpaid) position.
- Members of the Board of Trustees may have a financial obligation to the organization in case of financial disaster.

Trustees are usually elected on to the Board by other members of the company (some of whom are themselves volunteers) and will most likely have to produce and present their 'case' for election, providing personal and professional references and affidavits. Trustees are selected because of their proven commitment to the organization and/or because they have particular relevant skills to offer (e.g., management, medical, accountancy, and legal skills, etc.).

In some organizations, there is the opportunity to 'co-opt' board members. The purpose of this is to ensure a comprehensive skill mix and equitable representation of views of interested parties. However, these 'volunteers' may have very little previous knowledge of the work of the organization and what knowledge they have may not be detailed.

It is desirable that all Trustees have an induction programme the extent of which will in part depend on their previous involvement with the organization and their knowledge base. In the UK, over 70% of Trustees are from professional or intermediate occupations and in 1995, 66% did not receive any induction or training when they first became a Trustee.[6]

It is suggested that new Trustees attend the mandatory induction that all other new paid staff and volunteers attend. In addition there is a need for a Trustee-specific induction/education/training programme to explain the roles and responsibilities of Trustees and the board in relation to the hospice/palliative care service. When the individual needs of new Trustees are known a programme of induction can be tailored for their needs.

Training of Trustees is discussed in Chapter 5 but a Trustee is usually in post for a minimum of three years (depending on the organization's constitution), and they can have a big impact on the organization's management and policy.

Trustees working as 'ordinary' volunteers

If someone wants to work as an 'ordinary' volunteer as well as sitting on the Board of Trustees are there any questions that need to be addressed?

◆ How will the other volunteers feel about this?

◆ Can this volunteer act in an appropriate manner in their role as a non-Trustee volunteer? Has the volunteer's attitude changed since becoming a Trustee and will/does this cause conflict?

◆ How do the paid staff managing this volunteer feel?

◆ How do you, the VSM, feel? Do you feel you are able to manage this volunteer effectively?

Resentment and conflict can and do arise and the VSM must know how to tackle them.

Close relatives of salaried staff applying to be volunteers

A clear management policy is essential:

◆ What is the policy going to be and who decides it?

◆ Will it allow family members of paid staff to be accepted as volunteers or not? Will it allow family members of Board members/Trustees to become volunteers?

◆ What should an existing volunteer do when a family member becomes a paid member of staff or a Board member/Trustee? Should they discontinue volunteering (at least for the duration of the official appointment for Board members/Trustees)?

◆ How do you prevent nepotism—favouritism shown to family and friends?

The creation and adherence to this policy will once again be a reflection of the organization's senior management trust, support, and professional respect for the VSM.

Key issue: A clear policy needs to be in place about employing as a volunteer a close relative of a member of staff.

Documentation and data protection

Everything that the Volunteer Service Manager does should be according to clear and realistic standards and policies that are reviewed and audited regularly to ensure best practice and regulated by relevant data protection legislation.

It is useful to sign/initial and date any written entries and maintain a record of the names and position held of those who have the right to write in the paper or computer files in the volunteer services office. The list will record the person's full name and signature and initials to help with the identification of entries.

Records should be appropriate, relevant and succinct—monitored, and audited regularly (quarterly, half-yearly, annually) and unnecessary data regularly removed. Confidentiality must be maintained with access to records (paper or computer) limited to designated users using a security system (locked cabinet/password-protected). It is advisable to keep paper records for a minimum of six to eight years.

The volunteers must be aware of how and where their records are being kept. If these records are to be used for any mailing list, etc., by any one other than those in the organization then permission must be sought of the individuals. Volunteers are usually entitled access to their records.

In conclusion, the selection of volunteer staff is exercising a legal and moral obligation to choose the best and most appropriate people for your organization— to guarantee quality and safety. A robust, effective and equitable selection policy alongside a strong training and education strategy, will help to ensure that the common misunderstanding that 'voluntary' means 'amateur' does not persist.

Acknowledgement

The author wishes to acknowledge her indebtedness to Maggie Brain for her advice and help in preparing this chapter.

References

1. Smith J D (1997). Organising volunteers. In *Voluntary matters—Management and good practice in the voluntary sector*, (ed. P Palmer and E Hoe), pp. 277–302. Directory of Social Change, London.
2. Plain English Campaign. www.plainenglish.co.uk
3. McCurley S and Lynch R (1998). *Essential volunteer management* (2nd edn). Directory of Social Change, London.
4. Hudson M (1999). *Managing without profit—The art of managing third sector organisations* (2nd edn). Penguin, London.
5. Ford K (1993). *The effective trustee. Part One: Roles and responsibilities.* Directory of Social Change, London.
6. The Voluntary Sector National Training Organisation (2000). *Draft voluntary sector workforce development plan 2000.* www.nvco-vol.org.uk

Chapter 5

The training and education of volunteers

Purpose, aims, objectives, and outcomes

This chapter deals with training and education and although these terms are often used interchangeably they are subtly different.

Training is the act or process of teaching or learning a specified skill especially by practice. This equips the individual, for a specific task or role. The skills may be transferable but the outcome is quite discreet and measurable.

Education develops intellectual, moral, and social skills through systematic instruction and experience. It is a broader concept than training. It gives:

+ underlying knowledge;
+ philosophy;
+ understanding;
+ skills that can be used in a variety settings.

The outcome is a deeper level of understanding that is diffuse, transferable, and not always easily measurable.

What do volunteers expect from their training and education?

It must be recognized that individuals have very different expectations of their volunteering experience. Some people will think of themselves as a 'professional volunteer', those whose 'job' to them is being a volunteer but most will consider themselves as 'being there to help', usually in their spare time.

Whilst all volunteers look for job and personal satisfaction from their volunteer experience not everyone will want to take on responsibilities or 'develop', but for some volunteers educational opportunities and career development may be very important.

Volunteer work can be seen as:

+ a stepping-stone to paid work or full-time education/training;
+ an opportunity for free or reduced cost education and training;
+ an opportunity to try something different—learn new skills/new experiences;
+ an opportunity to consolidate prior learning/experience/skills;

- providing a work record/references;
- a positive employment attribute, the public and potential employers see volunteers as trusted and caring people (especially volunteers working in a hospice or palliative care setting (i.e. working with the dying is often seen as the epitome of 'good work'));
- a negative employment attribute, where people believe volunteer work is for those who would not be considered suitable for paid employment.

The differences between individual expectations of the volunteer role together with previous educational experiences means that the training/education provided can be seen in different ways, a perk, threatening, a necessary evil or as a great opportunity.

A good volunteer selection process along with clearly defined educational opportunities—that are of direct benefit to patient care whilst not being a barrier or threat to potential volunteers—will help to avoid exploitation or misuse of your voluntary service as a 'training agency' and ensure the recruitment of committed volunteers.

Why is it necessary to train and educate volunteers?

One of the main purposes of the education of all staff, including volunteers, is to ensure a *common minimum knowledge base* and a universal understanding of the philosophy, work, values and role of the organization.[1, 2]

Volunteer training/education is therefore provided to support patient care, to ensure standards of care and safe practice and to ensure appropriate public representation of the organization.

An introduction to voluntary service work will ensure that the key principles of palliative care are understood:[1]

- focus on quality of life;
- whole-person approach;
- care encompasses both the dying person and those who matter to that person;
- patient autonomy and choice;
- emphasis on open and sensitive communication.

It will ensure that no one is in any doubt as to what is expected of him/her regarding:

- confidentiality;
- professionalism;
- maintaining the organization's good image and reputation.

And will ensure:

- appropriate information and skills to ensure safe and best practice are imparted;
- which in turn will maintain quality and standard of work and care;

- will maintain and improve motivation;
- enable personal development;
- improve job satisfaction.

Additional/further training/education will help an individual's professional and personal development but it is also only through the training and education of staff that a service can grow and develop, its staff are a precious resource and should be nurtured. It must also be remembered that education is a two-way process, the organization can and must learn from its staff.[3]

The three elements of volunteer training/education
Statutory, mandatory, and voluntary: *Must*, *Should* and *Could*
Statutory: *Must*

Required by law—local and national employment law, Health and Safety laws, etc. These include:

- all new volunteers.
- updates to existing staff.
- role change/development.

The frequency and necessity of statutory training/updates requirements must be made clear to each volunteer, failure to attend training/updates will mean that they cannot work or continue to work in that role.

An example of statutory education/training is Moving and Handling (M&H)—a requisite of Health and Safety legislation and insurance. Every one *must* have comprehensive initial M&H training and then updates according to their role/risk (e.g. high, medium, low).

Mandatory: *Should*

Compulsory—a requirement determined by the organization. An organization will set minimum training standards/requirements that must be met in order for a volunteer to work in a specific role or area.

An example of mandatory education/training is the *induction* programme—this will be discussed in more detail later.

In addition to a general induction there are three distinct working areas/categories to consider.

1 *Non-patient areas*
- charity shops;
- donations transport—van drivers and assistants who collect donated items for resale in the charity shops.
- fund-raising.
- direct contact with the general public, which may includes some contact with patients and/or relatives including bereaved relatives.

2 *Patients and relatives contact areas*

- Home care.
- Day care (day hospice).
- In-patient area (bedded unit).
- Out-patient clinic (ambulatory clinic).
- Drivers for transport or patients.
- Coffee bar or restaurant staff.
- Bereavement support.
- Reception.
- Catering.
- Housekeeping, etc.

All volunteers may work within patient areas and will have prolonged, regular contact with patients and/or relatives, including bereaved relatives.

3 *Working in a professional capacity* (see also Chapter 12)

This includes working unpaid as:

- Nurse.
- Doctor.
- Physiotherapist.
- Hairdresser.
- Complementary therapist, etc.
- Trustee/Board Member.

These volunteers will need to produce evidence of relevant qualifications and registrations pertinent to their profession and may in addition need specific qualifications to work with patients with palliative care patients (e.g. lymphoedema massage). An example of mapping training/education requirements is shown in Table 5.1.

Voluntary: *Could*

Chosen to undertake for professional and/or personal development not a required element:

- to provide additional skills to enhance the volunteer role/job/experience;
- advanced learning (e.g. a counselling/or bereavement course), building on existing skills;
- unrelated to the volunteer role/job but will advance his/her personal skills and development (e.g. a computer course when working as a driver for patients, etc.). (Care must be taken regarding such payments in kind, and employment law—suggest volunteer pays for such training.)

Table 5.1 Volunteers: An example of training/education requirements.

Induction	Non-patient areas	Patients and relatives contact areas	Working in a professional capacity
Customer service/ communication skills	■		■
Finance/Cashier	■		
Fund-raising/Public liability/health and safety	■		
Bereavement	■		■
Clinical skills (e.g. feeding, bathing)			■
Use of equipment (e.g. hoists)	■		■
Drivers' training	■		
Basic first aid			
Food hygiene			
Disease information (e.g. symptoms, nutrition)			■
Task-specific training	■		■
Trustee induction			■
Trustee role-specific training			■

Resources

Time, money, appropriate trainers/educators, facilities, materials, and access

Before discussing in more detail the different programme options there are a number of issues that require some discussion as they can affect the how, where, when, and why of the training/education provision.

Time: What time is available to dedicate to training?

This will depend on:

- what the training is;
- who is conducting it;
- where they are conducting it;

but must include an element of preparation time.

- what time are volunteers prepared to give?
- will they be put off if they have to attend numerous days of 'unnecessary' classes before they can even start to help?

This can be a particular problem with those working in non-patient areas (e.g. charity shops; they may not see the need or significance of patient care details and communication skills).

Money: What money has been made available for training?

- Is there a training budget?
- Is it a separate budget for volunteer training or is it part of a larger training budget?
- Who administers the budget and who says yes or no to different training requests?
- Is any training charged?
- Is there money available for materials?
- Is there money available to buy in expertise?
- Is there money available to train people to teach or in subject specific skills (e.g. moving and handling)?

Appropriate trainers/educators: Who does the training?

- Does the organization have an education department or some paid lecturers?
- Are you (the Voluntary Service Manager) expected to do the training?
- Do you have the skills/qualifications to train/educate?
- Who can help you?
- Do you have to buy in the expertise?
- Which courses need specialists to conduct them?
- Dose the introduction/induction programme need specialist input (e.g. moving and handling, Health and Safety to meet legal requirements or recognized standards)?
- Is it appropriate to ask volunteers to help to train/educate?
- What happens with 'on the job training' who and how are the supervisors/trainers in these areas designated? (See the *Delivery* section.)

Facilities and materials: Do you have any dedicated training/education rooms?

- Are they of adequate size—how many people can attend induction training at any one time is the room registered under Health and Safety to cater for this number.
- Do you have to share facilities with other departments and are these rooms conducive to learning?
- Are they air-conditioned/heated/ventilated?
- Are there enough chairs; are they comfortable?
- What equipment is available—screen, whiteboard, flip chart, video, etc.

- Do you have to share this equipment; is this a problem?
- Where are the rooms and toilets located do they have disabled access, is there public transport available?
- What refreshments are available—how often, are they free?
- Do you take the training out to sites (e.g. charity shops)?
- Do you have or need appropriate videos about the organization, fire regulations, etc.?
- Do you have access to acetates, to a flip chart, paper, and pens?
- Are you going to supply handouts, workbooks or certificates?
- Who pays for printing and reprographics?

Access: Routes to and through training and education (see Fig. 5.1)

- The existing volunteer will be given the opportunity for appraisal/assessment that will include a training needs analysis (TNA) that will identify new courses, updates, and refresher courses needed or wanted.
- Pathways and competencies—certain courses or areas of study/training when achieved in a predetermined order will lead to a particular level of competency which in turn can lead to taking on a specific role or level of responsibility (e.g. team leader).

Planning

Purpose, content, and duration

For each course, lecture, pathway and competency the purpose, the content, the duration and the assessment must be decided:

- Who is this course/lecture aimed at, will there be a mixture of volunteers, paid staff, and Board Members/Trustees?
- Will there be a cultural mix?
- Will it be a very mixed age group?
- What educational, literacy, and ability levels will be present?
- What are the audience's motivations for learning?
- What level is the course (i.e. basic/introductory, intermediate, advanced)?
- Is the course a registered academic course (i.e. registered with an external awarding body or is it a non-academic course certificated for attendance/achievement by the organization only)?
- Is it a stand-alone lecture/course or part of a competency pathway?
- What and how will it be assessed?

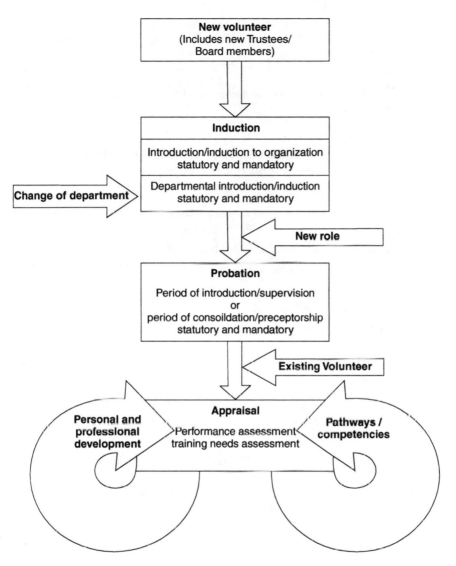

Figure 5.1 Volunteers' access to and through training and education.

Course information document (CID)

It will help to write a course information document (CID) (or course information form or file—CIF). The CID will help you to identify:

- What the content of the course should be.
- What the learners should be able to do with the skills and knowledge they have (i.e. what tasks will it enable them to undertake)?
- Under what conditions should the learners be able to use their knowledge and skills to perform these tasks?
- How well do they need to perform the tasks and how will this be judged?

The CID will also be a resource to others but it will change—it is a working document and will reflect the information and understanding at that time.

In the CID state:

+ The subject area experts (SAE) or subject matter experts (SME).
+ The course leader.
+ The teaching staff available.
+ The target audience—who and how many—it is useful to state a maximum and minimum number needed for the course to be viable.
+ The rationale—why is this course needed?
+ The aims—general statements that indicate the purpose and general outcome of this learning.
+ The objectives—more specific statements that will reflect the content.
+ The learning outcomes—what you hope the attendees will be able to do by the end of the course.

Indicative course content will state the:

+ subjects to be covered and content of each session—must reflect the 'need' not what would be 'nice';
+ time allocated for this session;
+ delivery method, the materials/facilities needed;
+ method of assessment of completion/competency (e.g. attendance, number of times completed, etc.).

If particular videos, books or exercises are used they should be clearly stated here indicating their length, and copies of teaching materials and handouts should be available.

The experts may be paid staff or volunteers (i.e. the best people to help draw up the CID/CIF). Volunteer involvement will help to:

+ encourage ownership;
+ provide motivation to other volunteers;
+ keep the content relevant.

An example of successful volunteer involvement was in training drivers for the transport of patients.

> Experienced volunteer drivers were asked to help put together a short training session for new drivers, which they were delighted to do. In conjunction with the Volunteer Service Manager, they created an induction pack that included a training session, a 'task' checklist, and a buddy system for new drivers and they then went on to develop support/training sessions at regular intervals.

Involvement like this will highlight to volunteers their importance to the organization and respect of their views, it encourages communication between all staff and helps team building.[4, 5]

Having completed the CID it is good practice to circulate it to all interested parties, that is, other staff and volunteers involved in the relevant areas for their comments as to its content and format, asking:

• Is it realistic?
• Does it reflect what is needed?
• Is it achievable?

Volunteers' involvement and comment is very valuable and will often highlight views and issues previously overlooked.

Delivery

This section discusses theories on learning, skills, attitudes, and knowledge required for successful delivery and the methods employed.

How do we learn?

Training and education is not just about learning a specific skill it is also an experience and should be a pleasant one. Learning is about change, a change in the way we see and think about the world around us and ultimately a change in how we interact with that world.

Volunteers working in palliative care will nearly all be adults and this fact should never be overlooked. When educating and training adults, their previous experience and knowledge must be acknowledged and valued,[8] building on what they already know and can do.

We all employ what we learn in different ways:

• *Activists* are people who like to get on and get going straight away—they do not wait for instructions or read the manuals.
• *Reflective learners* like to sit back and think a while, perhaps watch someone else before having a go.
• *Theorizing learners* want to put things into a logical step-by-step order to make a clear straightforward picture out of a lot of complex information.
• *Experimental learners* want to experiment, they want to find new and more effective ways of doing things and they may take shortcuts.

In adult education, our teaching must be flexible and varied enough to accommodate and support all learning styles whilst still achieving the predetermined aims, objectives and learning outcomes.

Skills, attitudes, and knowledge

What skills are needed to successfully deliver education and training to hospice volunteers? The following list of *Communication skills* has been developed from a list produced by Michael Meighan.[4]

• *Active listening*—awareness, understanding and attention:
  – body language,
  – non-verbal responses,

– appropriate verbal responses,

– summarizing,

– congruence.

♦ *Effective presentation*—to keep interest and provide clear information:

– language—concise, non-jargon,

– voice and eye contact—modulation and be inclusive.

Remember, you are speaking to inform and impress with the content rather than with yourself the speaker.

– use of equipment and aids—if you are using any audio or visual aids— (acetates, slides, etc.)—you must be familiar with the content and the order,

– look at content of audio visual aids—these should be relevant, concise and easy to read.

Proof read all written material.

Good organization, preparation, and administration can make life a lot easier for yourself and others and shows efficiency and reliability.

Ensure you, or those assisting you, have the knowledge required for the course:

♦ Self-awareness and self-knowledge—your own abilities, beliefs, prejudices, and values

♦ Theories on learning.

♦ Structuring a programme—training needs, content, aims, and objectives, delivery, etc.

♦ People and behaviour, special needs, cultural, social, and religious needs.

♦ The effects of stress—in particular the stresses that working in palliative care can create.

♦ Bereavement and loss theories.

♦ Group dynamics.

♦ Working with volunteers.

♦ The key principals of palliative care.

♦ Philosophy, purpose, work, and structure of the organization.

♦ Equity, equal opportunities.

♦ Appropriate national and international standards and legislation.

This is not a definitive list.

In addition, every group you encounter is comprised of individuals. In effect, you are managing a group of individuals and you will need to have or develop the following:

♦ people skills—friendly approachable,

♦ negotiating—respectful, adaptable, flexible,

♦ motivation—positive, encouraging, enthusiastic,

♦ problem solving—helpful, caring, determined,

♦ decision making—assertive, confident, reliable,

- selling—committed, realistic,
- observation—non-judgemental,
- questioning.

And at all times ensure confidentiality and keep a sense of humour.

Methods of delivery

Research and experience shows that we learn best through interaction and participation and retain 85% of the information supplied, whereas through listening (in a lecture) we only retain 5% of the information supplied.

Effective training/education will incorporate a number of delivery methods to ensure a varied programme that will make best use of resources and maintain interest. These will include:

- 'Show, tell, and do'.
- Didactic—lectures.
- Discussion.
- Role-play.
- Group work.

Group work helps 'break the ice' it gets people talking to each other and working together and if you are doing more than one group work exercise it is useful to get the people to swap around to form different groups each time—so making them talk and work with a different set of people.

- 'Show, tell, and do':[5]
  - shown either through the use of models or diagrams or by the teacher performing the task,
  - told the information,
  - doing—the student has a go.

Most often the telling and showing go together—'doing' is not always possible.

- *Didactic,* lectures are not very interactive and should be kept short and interspersed with activities. Support with written information.
- *Discussion* can work well but the group needs to 'gel' for this to work best. Discussion can be useful when looking at issues around confidentiality and boundaries.
- *Role-play* is very useful especially for communication skills but you will find that nobody (or very few) will want to take part—will work best with a group who have got to know each other a little.

Training/education programmes

The full training and education programme that is available to volunteers through your organization may be vast and there is not the space here to discuss the different variations that could be made available. However, it is worth considering what your organization's stance is regarding education and training as this attitude or commitment will determine what is provided, at what level and for what purpose.

A full range of training/education will include the basics for advanced courses, formal or informal learning, leading to a certificate of attendance, competency to perform a specific task or even a local or national qualification or certification. The training/education opportunities may be provided 'in house' but will also take advantage of external resources, including conferences, association/society, and committee membership. Volunteers should also be included in any organizational representation (e.g. ethics committees, awareness campaigns, etc.).

The learning experience should always be a positive one. One must not assume that an adult learner is an experienced learner; often, their last learning experience was many years ago at school and they may feel they have 'got out of the habit' or feel threatened just by the thought it. We have all had a bad education experience at some time in our lives (usually school) and these along with lack of motivation and boredom can be barriers to learning.

Learning must be recognized as an active process—it is interaction with a purpose.

Induction

A good induction is neither complex nor costly. It requires a clear and explicit process and good communication.[6]

Volunteer introduction/induction will be based around thanks and gratitude and around the 'must know', 'should know', and 'could know' of a new job/environment. All those engaged in the learning must feel valued, respected as an individual, needed, and welcomed—they are going to be an asset and complementary to the high quality service already provided.

Induction needs to be professionally informal—reflecting the ambience, hospitality, and atmosphere of the organization and its care. It must be a well-planned programme using good techniques. The involvement of different staff members in the delivery adds variety but also demonstrates team working and some friendly interdisciplinary banter helps to create a relaxed and friendly atmosphere. By employing a combination of 'teaching' staff—some of whom are clinical staff, and not primarily educationalists, can subliminally communicate an amazing number of messages.[7, 8]

The induction programme

The induction programme (it can also be called 'orientation') will include:[7, 8]

- Cause or organization orientation.
- System orientation.
- Social orientation.

Orientation: direction and bearings—finding one's way.

Cause or organization orientation: An introduction to the work of the organization

This includes:

- History.
- Description of the cause.
- The client group.
- Mission statement.
- Values and philosophy.
- Programmes and services.
- Future plans.

This will enable a conscious decision, an emotional and intellectual commitment to the basic purpose of the organization.

System orientation: An introduction to the organizational systems

This includes the volunteer management system. Use 'What would I like to know?' to draw up a list:

- The structure (management, hierarchy).
- Funding and fund-raising.
- Volunteer involvement in the organization:
  - roles,
  - responsibilities,
  - reporting/management,
  - policies and procedure.
- Facilities and equipment.
- Key activities.

Providing organizational context, where the volunteer fits in and where particular roles fit into the whole. It also enables the volunteer to understand the organization and so be an effective communicator on behalf of the organization.

Social orientation: Introduction to the organization's social community

This includes the staff, trustees, other volunteers—where the individual volunteer fits in. Some of this will take place as part of the departmental induction but the basics will be covered in the organizational induction:

- Introduction to colleagues.
- Introduction to support systems and to supervisors/mentors.
- Highlighting the benefits of volunteering for the individual.
- Looking at the opportunities available for growth and development.
- Reinforcing the value of their contribution.

An *accompanying written introduction pack* will include the organization's mission statement, philosophy, volunteering policy, moving and handling, health, safety, and fire policies (as bulleted lists) and contact information.

The generic induction you choose may be short and basic, or longer and more detailed and therefore will affect the content of any departmental induction.

Departmental induction

This can be seen as:

◆ part of the probation period;

◆ including mandatory training;

◆ specific to the needs of the department;

◆ devised between the manager and the volunteer;

◆ individual to that volunteer based on the job specification for that role.

Task-specific training/education

Those topics identified as 'task-specific' indicate that this is training to a level of competency in a specific task (e.g. patient feeding, using hoists). There will also be either a preceptorship (period of teaching or instruction) or a supervised period, whereby an individual will introduce the use of his/her skills clinically in a measured way. Each task will have minimum supervisory criteria associated with the competency. This supervisory/preceptorship period, or aspects of this period, can be increased to meet individual needs, at the request of the volunteer or their supervisor, to ensure that both parties feel confident and secure.

The 'qualified staff' involved in the procedure (this may include volunteer staff) and current legislation will determine the competencies of a task. Feedback from volunteer staff should be incorporated into decision making—often, the volunteers are the best people to be involved in drawing up training and competency initiatives.

Probation

Each volunteer will be allocated a mentor/supervisor by the manager of that department with whom they will meet regularly. It will be the responsibility of *both people* in this relationship not only to draw up and agree a probationary period timetable to include statutory and mandatory education and training, but also to ensure that these agreed goals are supported and met. A checklist of these criteria can be held by both parties and used as to ensure that the criteria are met (checked and signed) and that minimum time scales are adhered to (see Appendices).

The responsibility of successful completion of the probationary period lies with both parties. The mentor/supervisor relationship continues after probation and forms the basis for continued assessment and appraisal.

Evaluation

In order to ensure that your course is on track you need to evaluate it. Evaluation will involve feedback from the volunteers who will be given the opportunity to comment on the quality, the content, the delivery, and the usefulness of the course. At the end of each course an evaluation form should be completed by all attendees allowing comment on individual elements of the course and on the course overall.

Evaluation of outcomes will come from volunteer feedback but also through evaluation of the volunteer's knowledge and work once they are in a department via their mentor/supervisor/manager.

Some of the outcomes from induction or other courses are not going to be instantly apparent immediately after a course and will only become evident in time and after some experience. The mentorship, supervision, and preceptorship of volunteers that form part of their probation should provide feedback on how much they have taken on from the courses they have attended and how well they integrate that to their practice. This gives information on the progress of the volunteer but also to some extent, on the usefulness of the content and effectiveness of the delivery of a course. The volunteer at regular mentor/supervisor meetings will be asked to comment regarding their induction, and further training.

All feedback should be treated seriously and a method of collation and audit of this information should be in place. Similar suggestions received independently from a number of people, paid staff or volunteers should be acted on—which may mean adjustment to the content or delivery or assessment associated with a course. (See Figure 5.2.)

Standard setting and audit

This enables the value, content and outcomes of courses, competencies, and pathways to be determined, tested, and changed if necessary. It will also allow for changes in legislation, approach, and the recommendations of research. The setting of standards enables audit of quality and effectiveness and provides a minimum standard framework to adhere to.

Assessment

Most people hate the idea of assessment and are often intimidated by the idea that they are to be 'tested', but somewhere along the line a judgement has to be made as to the suitability of the volunteer to a job or environment.

Assessment recognizes achievement, identifies goals, and motivates.

Usually, volunteer assessment is seen as informal and non-threatening but some volunteers prefer a more formal approach so assessment of volunteers needs to be flexible and to meet the needs of the organization and of the volunteer. All organizations do some form of assessment.

Appraisal

Most organizations will have an appraisal scheme. Appraisal is a support mechanism and should not be used as a route for punishment. Volunteers' formal use

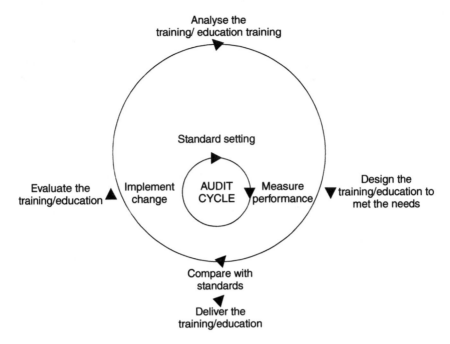

Figure 5.2 The training and audit cycle.[4]

of the appraisal scheme is usually optional: some may like to have formal feedback on their performance and the opportunity to put a training needs analysis together as previously discussed. Others feel threatened by this perceived 'judging' of their performance and prefer a more informal approach.

Continuous assessment is important for both the organization and the volunteer:

- Encourages volunteer involvement and motivation.
- Monitors performance and provides feedback on progress.
- Helps to ensure quality and maintenance of standards.
- Helps in shaping the volunteers future learning scheme—training needs analysis.

All assessments/interactions must be documented this will be especially important at times of conflict or discipline. Volunteers, like paid staff, are subject to and protected by the disciplinary and grievance procedures and legislation relevant to your organization.

The manager/team leader will give appropriate feedback to the Voluntary Service Manager when necessary—usually when there is a problem.

Training records

The holding of statutory, mandatory, and individual training records may be the responsibility of the Voluntary Service Manager, the education/training department or officer, or the volunteer himself/herself.

The planning, delivery, evaluation, and audit of the education/training provided can be the responsibility of the VSM or a designated education/training staff member or department.

Whatever system is in place or you choose to adopt, the following points are essential:

- Clearly state who is responsible for what—induction, probation, training, and appraisal.
- The staff involved in education, appraisal, supervision, mentorship, and preceptorship are suitably trained and supervised.
- Someone takes on the responsibility of holding the volunteer training records and ensures notification of statutory and mandatory updates
- The written minimum standards for induction/probation are being met and course content and competencies meet with local and national guidelines, insurance, and Health and Safety legislation.
- There is a reporting mechanism for problems/grievances.
- Evaluation is regularly conducted and the results utilized.

Training and education of Trustees

As stated in Chapter 4 on the selection of volunteers, Trustees are usually selected because of their proven commitment to the organization and/or because they have particular relevant skills to offer (e.g. management, medical knowledge, accountancy skills, etc.). Some Trustees will therefore be new to your organization and may have very little previous knowledge of the its work.

The responsibility for Trustees' education and training can vary from organization to organization. It may well be the responsibility of the VSM and/or the education officer/department especially where it overlaps with established courses, or it may be considered the sole responsibility of the Board and senior management.

It is preferable that some of the Trustees' induction would be conducted alongside other staff and volunteers to encourage openness, understanding, and team working. It is also advisable that any further educational requirements are devised/developed with educational staff/department input/advice.

Trustee induction should be based around:

- cause or organization orientation;
- system orientation;
- social orientation.

What do Trustees need in their induction?

In addition to attending the organization's normal introduction/induction an annual induction for new Board Members should be instigated. It must be acknowledged that some organizations will have insufficient new Trustees at any one time to justify running an annual induction session and so alternative induction programmes should be devised, for example, a workbook and individual sessions, or working with other similar organizations to provide a local or regional resource.[6]

Trustee-specific induction information

This comprises the following:

- The organization's constitution.
- The purpose and functions of the Board of Trustees—terms of reference for the Board and committees—powers and rules of governance.
- Specific Trustee roles and responsibilities—chair, vice chair, treasurer, other officers, etc., and as ambassador/representative of the organization to the public—codes of conduct.
- Confidentiality—particular responsibilities regarding Board/organizational activities.
- Boundaries—to also include work of the Board and work of the managers.
- Trustees' liabilities and protection.
- Management philosophy and methodology—basic management options and methodology, adopted by the organization, members/roles of the management team, staffing policy, etc.
- Clinical audit, clinical governance, and quality standards.
- Supervision/mentorship, grievance, and disciplinary procedures/policies.
- Funding/financial management.
- The law—constitution and local, national, and international legislation.
- Further education opportunities.
- Health and Safety responsibilities of the Trustees.

Specific Trustee skills/education/training

- Presentation skills
- Chair—responsibilities and duties.
- Vice Chair—responsibilities and duties.
- Meetings—committee process and purpose.
- Treasurer—finance/accounting information/skills (identified as the most frequently occurring knowledge gap for Trustees).[9]

The Board of an organization is a coalition of people from a variety of backgrounds who must work together; they will provide leadership and must add value and be of benefit to the organization. A Trustee/Board Member should at all times uphold the Nolan Committee's seven principles of public life:[10]

1 Selflessness.

2 Integrity.

3 Objectivity.

4 Accountability.

5 Openness.

6 Honesty.

7 Leadership.

The Nolan Committee[10] also recognizes the need to promote and reinforce standards of conduct of all those engaged in public life through guidance and training, including induction training.

Acknowledgement

The author wishes to acknowledge her indebtedness to Maggie Brain for her advice and help in preparing this chapter.

Appendix 1
Orientation checklist—Page 1

The example below is indicative only.

The first date refers to the date the mentor shows/discusses the item.

The volunteer's initials and date confirm that they have received and understood the information.

Volunteer's name: Mentor's name: Date attended induction: Date of first attendance in department:	Date	Mentor's initials	Date	Volunteer's Initials
Introduced to the staff—who's who				
Shown department layout				
Shown emergency exits				
Shown the location of fire alarm points				
Discussed their role in case of fire				
Shown how to use the telephone system				
How and who to telephone in case of an emergency				
Importance and procedure of taking accurate messages				
Reporting accidents—staff and patients				
Staff identification, signing in and security				
Reporting sickness and unavailability				
Health and safety procedures				
Moving and handling procedures				
Mentor, probation and appraisal systems				
Confidentiality (statement signed)				
Boundaries and reporting mechanisms				
'Job description' discussed				

Orientation checklist—Page 2

Summary of initial meeting with the volunteer discussing relevant skills, attributes, interests, and abilities the volunteer feels they can offer to the department:

Date: Mentor's signature:

Date: Volunteer's signature:

Please identify any areas of concerns or perceived problems:

Date: Mentor's signature:

Date: Volunteer's signature:

Please identify any particular support or special needs required:

Date: Mentor's signature:

Date: Volunteer's signature:

What additional mandatory training has been identified?

Date: Mentor's signature:

Date: Volunteer's signature:

Appendix 2
Mentor/Supervision record—Page 1

Volunteer's name:

Mentor's name:

Length of probationary period (e.g. 3 months):

Date probationary period begins:

Date probationary period will end:

Agreed frequency of review/supervision
  meetings (e.g. weekly for 4 weeks
  and then fortnightly) review
  frequency at end of probation period:

Date:

Mentor's signature: Volunteer's signature:

Was the probation period completed successfully?   YES/NO

If NO please briefly state reasons and action here:

Review of frequency of mentor/supervision meetings, date:

Please state changes to the schedule here:

Date of first annual appraisal (if requested):

Mentor/Supervision record—Page 2

Date of mentor/supervision meeting	Mentor's initials	Volunteer's initials	Comments

Appendix 3
Probation checklist—Page 1

Volunteer's name (V):

Mentor/supervisor's name (M):

Date probation begins:

Date probation ends:

Below is a list of agreed competencies to be completed during the probationary period.

Task details: (e.g. use of hoist)
Agreed competency pathway: e.g. 30 minute training session with mentor, observe use $\times$ 1, assisted in use $\times$ 1, supervised use $\times$ 2.

To be completed by:

	Training	M	V	Observed	M	V	Assisted	M	V	Supervised	M	V	Supervised	M	V
Date																

Volunteer feels confident and is deemed competent, date:

Mentor's signature: Volunteer's signature:

Task details:
Agreed competency pathway:

To be completed by:

	Training	M	V	Observed	M	V	Assisted	M	V	Supervised	M	V	Supervised	M	V
Date																

Volunteer feels confident and is deemed competent, date:

Mentor's signature: Volunteer's signature:

Probation checklist—Page 2

End of probationary period review meeting, date:

Was probation period successfully completed?   YES/NO

If NO please state reasons and agreed action here:

If YES were any further education / training needs identified?

Date:

Mentor's signature: Volunteer's signature:

References

1. National Council for Hospice and Specialist Palliative Care Services (NCHSPC), (1996). *Education in palliative care.* NCHSPC, London.
2. National Council for Hospice and Specialist Palliative Care Services (NCHSPC) (1997). *Making palliative care Better: Quality improvement, multiprofessional audit and standards.* Occasional Paper 12. Glickman M/Working Party on Standards. NCHSPC, London.
3. Hudson M (1999). *Managing without profit—The art of managing third sector organizations* (2nd edn). Penguin, London.
4. Meighan M (1995). *How to design and deliver induction training programmes* (2nd edn). Kogan Page, London.
5. Forsyth I, Joliffe A, and Stevens D (1999). Delivering a course—Practical strategies for teachers. In *Lecturers and trainers* (2nd edn). Kogan Page, London.
6. The Ford Partnership and Help the Hospices (2000). *The trustee induction pack—The twenty-minute guide to being a hospice trustee.* Help the Hospices, London.
7. McCurley S and Lynch R (1998). *Essential volunteer management* (2nd edn). Directory of Social Change, London.
8. Smith J D (1997). Organising Volunteers. In *Voluntary matters—Management and good practice in the voluntary sector,* (ed. P Palmer and E Hoe), pp. 277–302. Directory of Social Change, London.
9. The Voluntary Sector National Training Organisation (2000). *Draft voluntary sector workforce development plan 2000.* http://www.nvco-vol.org.uk
10 Her Majesty's Stationery Office (HMSO) (1995). *The Nolan Committee's first report on standards in public life.* HMSO, London.

Chapter 6

The support of volunteers

Hospices and palliative care units, especially in the UK, have large volunteer teams to give help to the staff and enhance the environment of the organization. These individuals come to offer their time and skills for various reasons and their level of commitment and dedication is very special. Whoever they are, whatever they do, however long they work for the palliative care service, they need to be offered appropriate support. This chapter will address this challenge.

It is important that volunteers are satisfied in their duty, enjoy the experience and their attachment to the organization and, as a consequence, stay with the organization for some time. The introduction of a volunteer service has to be based on a well-planned, well-budgeted for, policy and programme which set out, from the first interview of the prospective volunteers to the time they leave the service, how they and the service will be managed.

This chapter will suggest ways in which volunteers will need to be supported in their time within the organization. The main text will be taking the 'career' of the volunteer from beginning to end in chronological order discussing at the different stages how this support might be delivered.

Introducing a volunteer service
Volunteer staff policy

Volunteers can be supported even before they present themselves for interview by the fact that a *Volunteer staff policy* is in place.[1] This lays out how the organization intends to manage, protect, and support their volunteers during their time on the lists. It is not only an important document for the volunteers, but also is important for the organization because any outside agency which intends to provide funds may well wish to see or know that such a document is in place. It is also considered to be best practice to have such a document. It will contain the different elements of care, support, and supervision necessary to ensure a happy, satisfied volunteer group. This will then result in a high volunteer retention rate which is the goal of any Volunteer Service Manager.

Support at the interview stage of a prospective volunteer

It is crucial that the interview and selection process for volunteers is effective for the organization and the individuals concerned. Supporting a volunteer should begin here at this first stage of their application to join the service (see Chapter 4).

Support before the first time on duty

Some organizations prefer their new volunteers to have attended an *induction/ orientation/education course* before they start their duties. All these terms are used to describe such a course. These can be useful in some areas such as one-to-one buddy volunteering with a client or patient. In this situation volunteers need information, help, and support before starting their duties.

There are both advantages and disadvantages of providing courses *before* a volunteer starts.

Advantages:

- Volunteers will meet other new volunteers at the course.
- Volunteers may feel better prepared and more comfortable to come into the unit to carry out their tasks.
- They may have had a chance at the course to listen to and speak to an experienced volunteer. This can be a very positive experience to new volunteers.

Disadvantages:

- Such courses can only be organized on a regular basis every four to six months because staff members are usually involved and so volunteers may have to wait until completing a course before starting regular duties. This wait can result in the volunteer becoming impatient and seeking another organization.
- Volunteers may feel less comfortable about helping in palliative care because they are only hearing about but not experiencing the special ambience that all units have.
- The success of the course depends considerably on the content and those who deliver it in order to maintain the interest of the new volunteers before they have experienced the area for themselves.
- Volunteers who have not had experience of courses or education sessions may be put off because they believe it is too formal an approach. All they wish to do is give their time to a good cause.
- Volunteers who have had experience of courses, seminars, and education sessions during their working life may not want to have to take part in these kinds of meetings just to become a volunteer.

Providing courses within six months of the new volunteer starting duty for a few weeks also has its advantages and disadvantages.

Advantages

The new volunteer has come to know the unit and some of the staff and feels comfortable about coming in to the course. They:

◆ meet other new volunteers who have just joined;

◆ have not had to wait to get started on their duties. Motivation is very important and it is good for new volunteers to start working as soon as possible;

◆ have some knowledge of the work and come with questions to the sessions and an eagerness to learn more about palliative care.

Disadvantages

◆ They may have not had the knowledge or confidence gained from a course to support the staff in the correct way even though their on-duty training has been carried out;

◆ They have not had the awareness and understanding of palliative care developed by the content of the courses before they start.

However, the courses are offered, they are essential to develop the knowledge, interest and awareness of new volunteers.

Support on the first day of duty

Support at this stage is primarily about being warmly welcomed into the unit preferably by someone the new volunteer has already met, usually the Voluntary Service Manager (VSM). The volunteer should have been given some background reading about the unit before coming in for the first time. This helps with the understanding of palliative care and how the particular unit cares for its patients and families. The next important step is to give them a short induction/ orientation programme.

Volunteers come in with great enthusiasm to start their duty but the first visit can be a daunting time for some new volunteers who may be anxious about it for many reasons.

◆ Will it be a sad place?

◆ Who will I be working with and will I like them?

◆ How will I feel when I go through these doors into the ward area?

◆ Will I manage to control my emotions if I see unexpectedly someone I know ?

◆ Can I cope with the Charity Shop till!

◆ Will there be help nearby if I have a problem?

◆ Am I at risk from these hospital infections I hear about?

◆ What will I get out of this commitment of time?

◆ Will I find satisfaction in this duty?

◆ Do I really have the skills that are needed in this area of palliative care?

All of these kinds of questions need to be addressed in the induction programme by the VSM and will be answered after the *probationary period* has been fulfilled (see below). It is likely that since the successful interview the new volunteer has had time to think about the task taken on and will need reassurance at this early stage.

The probationary period (see also Chapter 5)

The new volunteers will know before they come in for their first day of on-duty training that a *probationary period* is a necessary part of the initial phase of their time with the organization. This support mechanism should be written into the voluntary staff policy and should apply to all volunteers no matter which area they have chosen to help the organization. This period should extend over the first three or four months and it is a most important time because it is often found that people who volunteer for a palliative care unit do not really know how they will react to the environment.

At the end of this probationary period, a volunteer agreement/commitment will be discussed and signed by the VSM and the volunteer. This formalizes the volunteer as an established member of service. It also gives the volunteer an opportunity to discuss aspects of their duties which have not been easy for them. Of course, volunteers should always be informed of the 'open door' policy of the volunteer services office. This gives them freedom at any time to bring anxieties or questions to the attention of the volunteer office staff in the early days.

The commonest problems volunteers mention at this stage are:

- *They have difficulties with the volunteer(s) with whom they share the duty.* The answer is to try to find another 'slot' in the timetable for them. Keep a note that they should not be with this person if it can be avoided.

- *The timing is difficult for them.* Offer another duty time or another duty at a more convenient time.

- *The duty is fine in the summer but not in the winter because of dark evenings.* Offer a day-time slot if possible or arrange a lift home in the winter. Seasonal volunteers can be awkward to manage unless they are prepared each time they go 'on sabbatical' to join a new area or duty on their return.

- *They find the cash till too awkward to handle.* Offer them another duty.

- *They find the duty too boring. They need to be kept busy and the duty can be dull at times.* Again, offer another duty at a busier time.

- *They seem to be lacking the same enthusiasm or motivation with which they applied to help.* It may be that the organization is not for them. They must be given the chance to share this with the VSM and walk away to another organization if nothing can be done to retain their gift of time.

The VSM must give time and effort to this part of the individual support of new volunteers. It is crucial that in such a caring environment the volunteers feel that they themselves are cared for. They might find themselves unable to offer good care if their expectations as a volunteer are not fulfilled.

The new volunteer must know how to get help, how to contact the person in charge of their area, and at all times to feel able to contact staff from the volunteer office. The induction session could emphasize this information. This kind of support helps to make the new volunteer feel that they are part of the team, reduces anxiety, and gives a good impression of the care and support to come in the months, possibly years ahead as they help in the organization.

The first spell of duty will involve *training* for the specific task the volunteer has undertaken. This training is usually delivered by an experienced volunteer (see Chapter 5).

On the day of their first duty *after* training the new volunteer should not be left alone but be accompanied and supported by an experienced volunteer for company and advice. Most volunteers enjoy the company of others and for some this can be the main reason for applying to become a volunteer. Duties that can isolate them in a room or area where there is little contact with other people can be difficult to sustain. Those who take on such duties will possibly need more support and attention than those who are together in a small team on a regular basis.

Support through training, documentation, and education sessions (see Chapter 5)

The details of training very much depend on the work the volunteer will do: How much they need and how long it will be required are matters for each organization to evaluate. A good 'rule of thumb' would be that the closer a volunteer is likely to be to patients or relatives, and especially if they are actually working with patients, then the more rigorous the training they will need.

One method of supporting a volunteer who is very interested in being close to patients is to allow the volunteer to spend at least six months carrying out more routine tasks, such as in the coffee shop or flower room, before they move into patient care. This gives the volunteer time to get to know and understand the organization and how it operates and consequently gain confidence. It also gives the VSM and staff in the area concerned time to get to know the volunteer—this helps with selecting the appropriate volunteers for those teams that offer duties that involve working closely with patients.

Induction pack for volunteers

Providing a new volunteer with documentation in the form of an induction pack is an essential means of early support. Much information is given in the first phase of joining the volunteer service and it is unlikely that most volunteers will retain everything that is explained to them. Giving them written information about their duty is most useful and serves as a reference for them when queries do arise.

This induction pack can contain items such as:

◆ A letter of welcome.
◆ A brief history of the unit and the services it offers.

- A floor plan of the unit.
- Information on health and safety.
- A list of the many roles undertaken by volunteers in the palliative care service.
- Guidelines for the particular role the volunteer is being asked to undertake.
- Information about the processes in place for continuing support for volunteers (perhaps mentioning details of the probationary period, the first anniversary review, the service medals/badges given to volunteers after a certain number of years service, etc.).
- The volunteer commitment/agreement and what it contains.
- Emergency procedures in the event of fire and accident
- A copy of the volunteer staff policy.
- An illustrated guide to the staff uniforms to help them identify staff categories.

Ongoing training and education (see also Chapter 5)

Continuing education and update sessions are a necessary part of support. They keep the volunteers up to date with developments of the organization and its environment and help them to maintain a sense of confidence in what they are doing.

Update sessions are opportunities for volunteers to learn more about the hospice/palliative care service, to hear about new developments, to get information about changed routines, to meet new members of staff. They are invaluable for many reasons, for example:

- They help the volunteers to feel valued and part of the bigger team as they respond well to having staff explain and talk to them about the staff's own needs.
- They provide a means of communication with the staff. This contact should be encouraged in these sessions as it helps greatly with relationships between staff and volunteers which is vital for happy, productive teamwork.
- They give volunteers an opportunity to talk to staff and ask questions regarding their duties. Occasionally, volunteers might make suggestions which will, ultimately, help not only the staff and volunteers working alongside them but also the patients.

It cannot be emphasized enough that members of staff have a great part to play in helping volunteers to remain motivated and satisfied to stay in their duty for long periods of time. Working with and caring for volunteers should be built in to staff training and should be monitored carefully. Volunteers do not need and should not expect to be fussed over in their duties, but they should be acknowledged when they are around the unit and thanked occasionally by the staff.

Ongoing support

The organization that is supported by volunteers needs to support them in many ways as they go about their duties. Volunteers should not only be shown how much they are appreciated. They should know of the many things that have been put in place for them as well as for the staff.

♦ **Insurance.** They should be reassured that there is adequate cover to protect them and the organization. (This is discussed in Chapter 13.)

♦ **Out-of-pocket expenses.** On joining the service, volunteers should be told that these are available to ensure that anyone who feels that they are unable to afford to come in to help will not be disadvantaged. This is usually paid in arrears on presentation of a receipt.

♦ **First anniversary of joining the volunteer service.** On this anniversary, no matter how often the VSM has seen the volunteers in the preceding year, it is good practice to meet with the volunteers to thank them for their year's effort and to ask if they have any ideas, suggestions or problems to discuss. These times of being with a volunteer and listening to their comments are of great value and again reaffirms that they are part of a caring supportive team.

♦ **Annual informal meetings.** Ideally, the VSM should meet each volunteer, not only on the first anniversary, but on an annual basis. However, in most palliative care units and hospices where volunteer numbers are large this is not always possible or practicable. Even if such meetings are less frequent, say every two or three years, they are valuable for both the volunteer and the VSM.

♦ **Team meetings and update education sessions** as described above are important ways of bringing volunteers together.

♦ **Occasional social occasions.** There is no doubt that such events can be most enjoyable and are occasions when volunteers who might not otherwise see each other can do so in relaxed informal settings. However, much thought needs to be given to them and their cost. Many hospices and some palliative care units are run on a charitable basis and care must be taken, when 'entertaining' volunteers or rewarding them for their efforts, that the events which are held are not extravagant. Volunteers generally do not want to have the organization spend money on them to say 'thank you' so this aspect of support needs to be sensitively handled. Many units find the best times to run them are at Christmas or during 'Volunteer's Week' (UK).

♦ **Long service awards.** Many units offer their volunteers some sort of reward, be it a certificate or a brooch or a small medal they can wear when on duty. The first is usually awarded after five years service, then every five years thereafter. Each period of five years is marked either by a different brooch or a 'bar' to the medal. This is usually very acceptable to volunteers and if the award is a special badge they wear it with pride and indeed look forward to receiving it at a modest social occasion where the presentation is made by someone as important as the Chairman of the Trustees or a local dignitary.

♦ **Special events.** Some palliative care units and hospices recognize special birthdays, anniversaries, and the retirement dates of retired volunteers by sending cards or even flowers. Obviously, this recognition usually depends on the time the volunteer was with the organization and can be formally set out in the volunteer staff policy.

♦ **Christmas and festivals.** Depending on whatever are the local festivals and holidays such as Christmas, Passover, and New Year, volunteers can be sent a card or invited to a social event to mark these occasions

♦ **Cards or flowers.** Volunteers who become sick or bereaved should be sent a card or flowers from the volunteer office. A visit from a member of the volunteer office staff may also be considered. This kind of recognition during difficult times is always much appreciated.

♦ **Volunteer service newsletter.** This is an excellent way of communicating with volunteers. It gives added interest in the organization as volunteers can be kept aware of any new developments, such as new members of staff, additions to the buildings, and any news with particular relevance to the volunteer service itself, such as dates of events in the months ahead, newcomers to the service, and thanks to those who are leaving. Volunteers can be encouraged to contribute to such a publication and this adds to the interest and the content of the newsletter. This newsletter could be published twice a year in-house at little cost if a computer and efficient printer are available.

Volunteer team leaders/co-ordinators

The larger organizations can benefit from a *volunteer team leader/co-ordinator* (*TLC*) system to help with the management of rotas and help with other events such as the orientation, induction, and training of volunteers (see Chapter 3). This system not only gives support to the VSM but also is another interesting way of supporting volunteers by providing a 'promotion' for those who are able and wish to become more involved in the management of the volunteer service (see Chapter 3).

This system has to be carefully organized and managed by the VSM with the selection of the TLCs being of utmost importance.[2] These volunteers along with the volunteers who have been selected to provide training for new volunteers will need an extra level of support from the VSM.

Regular meetings with the VSM should take place with all who help with such tasks. It is recommended that these meetings should take place at least every two months. A social aspect can be built in here by having a meal together in the unit on the day of the meeting. This is a useful way of valuing those volunteers who take on the extra responsibility of helping the VSM in managing and training the volunteers.

Obvious as it sounds all volunteers should be offered a cup of tea or coffee during their time on duty and if they spend more than five hours in a day helping, then a meal also should be made available.

General support measures

It is important that the environment where the volunteers carry out their duties is adequately equipped. There should be available:

+ *Notice boards*, with space dedicated to the volunteer services if it is a board for staff and volunteers, or a board in the volunteer office for information, the rosters for the different teams, and special notices.
+ Appropriate *equipment* for the different duties done by volunteers, well maintained and simple to use and understand.
+ *Protective clothing* should always be available with clear instructions for *infection control procedures, hygiene* and any other protective measures required by the organization.

Much of this will be written in the Health and Safety handbook discussed in Chapter 13 on legal issues.

One of the most important and effective ways of supporting volunteers, as well as seeing them regularly, is to maintain an *open door policy*. Volunteers must know and understand that at any time volunteer office staff are available if a volunteer wants to see them. This contact is vital for teamwork and for giving confidence and trust in their support system.

Care must be taken not to abuse or take unfair advantage of the specially committed and flexible people that all volunteer services have on their lists. Enthusiastic offers of help will soon wane if a volunteer is asked to do too much too often. This over-use of a volunteer can upset the balance of what is given and what a dedicated volunteer receives. Especially in palliative care, volunteers should not become too involved with the patients and families as this can lead to a stressful time of loss for the volunteer when the patient dies.

Relationship with the VSM

In supporting volunteers during their time in a unit the most important thing is the relationship the volunteer has with the VSM and others who are connected with the volunteer service. The better that relationship is the better the service will run. Individuals who manage volunteers need to be very interested in each volunteer. They must remember (not necessarily write down) details of their volunteers' lives. The author would suggest that to store information about what has been called 'Grandchildren, Gran Canaria and Gall bladders' in one's memory can be very valuable. Such details about the families, the holidays, and the health of volunteers are not intrusive but can make a volunteer feel valued and important to the organization. When made to feel special this helps them to appreciate their part in the larger team and in turn enhances their commitment and their sense of being wanted and appreciated.

Support when a volunteer is in difficulty

Volunteers who suffer crises in their lives need to be supported through them. This does not mean that the VSM needs a certificate in counselling, but should display a calm approach, have a kindly listening ear, and be available and approachable.

In the case of *personal bereavement* it is necessary for volunteers to take time out until they feel ready to come back to help. This need not be dealt with in a formal way. In the author's experience volunteers who feel well supported are keen to come back sooner rather than later because of that support. They must feel comfortable to come back into the palliative care environment and it is the responsibility of the VSM to ensure that they do. The VSM will keep closely in touch with a bereaved volunteers and eventually the sign will be given that they wish to come back to their duties. At this point, the VSM should invite the volunteer into his/her office to talk about how he/she feels about their loss and what support the volunteer feels may still be needed to help he/she to adjust. If there is doubt about the readiness to come back then volunteers should be urged to take more time; perhaps come in occasionally to help with duties, such as preparing mail shots, where they are not exposed to the nursing area of the unit. This can help the adjustment process. This support is always much appreciated and allows volunteers to come back to their own duties at the appropriate time, a time that varies from individual to individual. This examination of their wish to come back is a crucial process that must be gone through by the VSM. Very rarely a volunteer, having suffered a sad loss, will decide that the palliative care environment is not suitable for him/her and will withdraw. This wish must be respected.

In the event of *illness*, either of a physical or mental nature, of a volunteer, he/she must be equally well supported. In palliative care, many volunteers first apply to join the volunteer service in middle age and may remain with the organization for many years. It is possible that not only can physical illnesses develop and affect their ability to work, but conditions, such as dementia, may occur. Unlike other conditions, sufferers may not be aware of the changes in their behaviour. The author has experienced four cases in seven years in post and has some suggestions how to deal with this situation.

Dementia is progressive and when it is first suspected then staff and team leaders should be alerted and be made aware of difficulties that may arise. The time will come when the volunteer will need to be 'counselled out' of the organization. This can be hard to achieve without distress to everyone concerned. One method of dealing with this difficulty is by involving the family of the affected volunteer. A letter or telephone call or a meeting with the family giving reasons why a demented family member should not return to his/her volunteer duties is necessary. This contact is swiftly followed by a visit to the volunteer by the VSM with a basket of flowers or other suitable gift, and a 'thank you' letter. This usually works well.

There can be a situation where there is no family support in which case the general practitioner (GP) may need to be involved. This needs the permission of the volunteer and requires to be approached sensitively. Managing a volunteer with such a condition can be delicate but must be handled decisively to protect the volunteer and the organization from a difficult and possibly dangerous situation.

Any condition whether physical or mental which causes the volunteer to be unable to carry out his/her duties effectively must be addressed by the VSM. This can be done by the VSM inviting the volunteer to come to the office to discuss his/her position in the volunteer team. It may be that permission needs to be given for the VSM to approach the GP of the volunteer to find out more about the case. Kindly dealing with this situation can support the volunteer as he/she moves out of his/her present duty, but not necessarily out of the organization altogether. It may be possible to find tasks that are more suitable to the volunteer's ability. This solution is good for the organization, the volunteer service and the volunteer.

Volunteers who steal, abuse drugs or alcohol or, in any way, do not obey the rules or procedures of the unit must be dismissed immediately. This is an obvious statement but crucial to observe to support everyone else who is involved with the organization. This is especially required for the other volunteers who have duties alongside the offending volunteer. Such procedures will be part of the volunteer staff policy.

Support for volunteers when they leave the organization

In every palliative care unit where so many volunteers are involved in many duties, there is always some turnover throughout the year. This is to be expected, acknowledged and accepted as normal. It is useful for the VSM to offer an exit/retiral questionnaire to be completed by volunteers when they have left their duties. The benefits of this are:

- It allows the volunteer to legitimately offer reasons why they are leaving.
- An opportunity is given to state whether or not they felt supported during their time in the organization.
- To hear from the volunteer about the enjoyable and satisfactory experiences of their voluntary work.
- It gives the VSM a sight of criticisms of the service. There is then a possibility of improving the service for all concerned.

Feedback of whatever nature is important when dealing with so many different individuals. The VSM and the staff concerned should always be trying to improve the quality of the volunteer service to the organization.

It can be difficult to get good, regular feedback from these questionnaires as the volunteer is not required to complete it as part of their commitment, but it is worth trying.

If a volunteer retires because they are unhappy or feel badly dealt with then this must be taken very seriously. The VSM should follow up all aspects of the case to discover what has been happening and take steps to comfort and support the volunteer in their anxiety. There can be many reasons for such a situation and the truth must be uncovered if the credibility of the volunteer service is not to be undermined. In general, volunteers are very loyal and will leave an organization rather than make a stand against poor treatment or conditions. It is important for the reputation of the organization and its standing in the community that such problems are addressed and volunteers are able to retire with some support for their case. It could be of course that the volunteer management itself is the cause of stress to volunteers. This must be addressed and dealt with by the line manager of the VSM.

Everyone in the organization should appreciate that volunteers, whether few or many, are an unofficial public relations group. They go out into the community with plenty to say about the organization and what they say has to be good. Supporting and valuing volunteers properly can have considerable benefits for the unit in attracting people and funds to the organization. The volunteers take their experiences outside and tell of the quality of care, for patients, relatives, staff and volunteers, for which palliative care is renowned.

Support for the VSM

This is a crucial issue for any volunteer service. Volunteers are more likely to be well managed if the VSM is well managed and supported. Most palliative care units now appreciate the value of a dedicated volunteer manager who is paid, has a budget, is responsible for the volunteers in his/her care and is accountable to the Board of Management for the service. Secretarial support should be available as well as an office and adequate computer equipment with a user-friendly database. The VSM should have regular access to senior members of staff to discuss volunteer matters with them, ideally as a member of the senior management team (see Chapter 3). This helps to pre-empt any difficulties that may arise between staff and the volunteer service.

Conclusion

Volunteers come to help in palliative care units for many reasons. They bring a wide range of skills and personal qualities and come form all parts of the social spectrum.

Resources are needed to introduce, manage, and retain these good people. The VSM must know his/her volunteers well and must encourage the staff of the organizations to be sensitive, appreciative, and value the role played by the volunteers.

There is no better feeling for a VSM than knowing a volunteer team is happy in its duty, is supported and appreciated by the staff involved and is giving dedication and commitment to the palliative care service.

This willing and generous gift of time to a hospice or palliative care unit by a large group of volunteers is one of the things that sets these places apart from other hospitals or care homes. They give invaluable assistance to the staff and they help create the special environment of peace and comfort appreciated by so many patients and relatives. To achieve the optimal results volunteers must themselves be fully and effectively supported.

References

1. McCurley S and Lynch R (1998). Appendix B. In *Essential volunteer management* (2nd edn), p. 211. Directory of Social Change, London.

Recommended reading

Adirondack S and Sinclair Taylor J (2001). *The voluntary sector legal handbook* (2nd edn). Directory of Social Change, London.

McCurley S and Lynch R (1998). *Essential volunteer management* (2nd edn). Directory of Social Change, London.

Chapter 7

Volunteers working in a comprehensive palliative care service

The experience on which this chapter is based was gained from initiating, developing and managing a palliative care volunteer service in a public hospital (or 'medical centre' as it is now more commonly called) in Australia. It had had an active volunteer service for four years before a palliative care service was started.

The author's previous experience includes many years of co-ordinating volunteers in other types of services before moving into palliative care.

What is a comprehensive palliative care service?

A comprehensive hospice/palliative care service is one with in-patient beds, a hospital palliative care team working in an acute hospital, and a community palliative care service or a close working association with one. Often, it also includes a day centre (sometimes termed a day hospice), both educational and research facilities and usually a bereavement service.

The hospital on which this chapter is based is a public (government-run) one which also has a university research area. The hospital facilities are divided into four sections one of which is the cancer section where the volunteer service is based.

The palliative care team provides care/consultancy services to:

- cancer wards;
- cancer out-patients (ambulatory) visiting the hospital;
- palliative care patients throughout the hospital, whether or not they have a malignant disease;
- palliative care unit with 20 beds;
- liaison with domiciliary/home based palliative care services (now usually referred to as a community palliative cares service).

The palliative care service is based in the cancer section of the hospital but its staff provide care and advice throughout the whole hospital.

The palliative care service

The palliative care consultancy team consists of:

- the medical director of palliative care;
- a nurse consultant co-ordinator of palliative care;
- medical officers;
- consultant palliative care nurses;
- social workers;
- pastoral carers;
- dietitians;
- physiotherapists;
- occupational therapists;
- manager of palliative care volunteer service (VSM);
- palliative care volunteers.

The other dimension of the service is the 20-bed palliative care unit, which has a designated nurse unit manager and its own palliative care nursing staff, the VSM, and the palliative care volunteers. The VSM and her assistants have offices near the palliative care unit.

A comprehensive palliative care service, like any palliative care service, provides holistic care for patients with life-threatening, incurable illnesses, and for their families and friends. The nurse co-ordinator of palliative care and the palliative care nurses are consultant nurses for the whole hospital.

They visit the patients, advise the staff, especially about pain control, and arrange for the patients' discharge from the acute wards to the palliative care unit, to a nursing home, to their own home, or to some other place of residence. Part of this discharge is organized with palliative care staff from a community-based palliative care service who will visit the patient at home. The staff of the hospital palliative care service liaise regularly with the community palliative care staff about patients they have in common, the former having got to know them when they were in-patients and the latter when they came back into the community for continuing care.

This chapter is about volunteers in the hospital and its palliative care unit settings but it should be noted that the community palliative care services also have volunteers who visit patients at home. The two groups of volunteers as with the staff complement one another.

Volunteers

Why have volunteers in a comprehensive palliative care setting?

In this hospital, it was decided to appoint a VSM to initiate a palliative care volunteer service because the palliative care and other staff felt that the patients needed more holistic care than they had time to give. They knew that someone taking time to just 'be there', to spend time with the patients was an important part of the patients' care and well-being. Unfortunately, funding is never enough to cover all needs so volunteers were looked at as a solution.

Which conditions govern the work of volunteers?

> **Key point**: It must be stressed that volunteers complement but never supplement the clinical management of other team members or members of staff (see later in this chapter).

Volunteers may never do anything that is part of any staff member's job description. The VSM must not ask a volunteer to do a task that would contravene this agreement with unions and staff. Volunteers are only allowed to work up to 16 hours per week in this hospital.

Although, as mentioned above, it was initially envisaged that volunteers would save precious hospital funds they do not do so directly but indirectly. They help to make the patient feel better cared for thus making the hospital run more smoothly and effectively. Another reason volunteers are welcome in a hospital and hospice setting is that they bring to the patient's bedside some of the outside world. The patients see nurses, doctors, and other professionals all day long and quite often feel vulnerable because they are the only person who is not a medical professional.

Volunteers are never paid a wage but may be reimbursed out-of-pocket expenses (e.g. petrol money for driving a patient, or for further education or training).

Volunteers may never give an opinion on anything medical.

How to describe a volunteer

The volunteer is someone who:

- like the patient, is not a health care professional;
- is not in a uniform but in normal everyday clothes;
- is a mother, father, sister, brother, husband or wife, just like the patient;
- has time to listen;
- is willing to just be there giving his/her undivided attention to the patient;
- can do little tasks for him/her;
- can listen to the patient's worries or who will talk about anything but illness if that is what the patient chooses;
- will take the patient for a walk even in a wheelchair;
- will help with meals;

◆ will help with grooming;

◆ always respects confidentiality.

In other words, a palliative care volunteer is a person who comes to see the patient with the *specific intention of doing what the patient wants him/her to do* within volunteer guidelines (see the Appendix).

Palliative care volunteers are part of the interdisciplinary palliative care team and must act and expect to be treated with respect as are all members of the team, both paid and unpaid.

What do volunteers do?

Each working day, the volunteers come to their office, sign on, and read the patient notes written in the daily workbook on the previous day. They then report for duty to the nurse unit manager (sister in charge) of the area in which they are working. Two volunteers work in each area, visiting patients separately from each other.

There are different times of duty and several different areas in which the palliative care volunteers work with the patients. They are:

◆ Day roster

◆ Palliative care unit

◆ Radiotherapy

◆ Evening roster

◆ 'One-to-one' (1/1)

◆ Specialized work

◆ Office work

◆ Fund-raising

The aim is to have each volunteer on day roster once a week and in the palliative care unit once a week for about four to six hours each time. The volunteers prefer to keep to the same two days each week but are happy to go where needed at these times.

There are many different volunteers working in our hospital (e.g. fund-raising, canteen, drivers, in the accident and emergency unit), and on some of the other wards as well as the palliative care unit. Each group of volunteers must attend a specialized education programme *before* working in the hospital

The Volunteer Service Manager always has the final say on what the palliative care volunteer is permitted to do.

Recruitment of volunteers

A person who has had cancer or any debilitating disease needs to discuss it with the co-ordinator of volunteers (or VSM) when applying to become a palliative care volunteer. The general rule is 12 months free of illness after the last appointment with a doctor.

The 12 months rule also applies to a prospective volunteer who has had a close relative or friend die. Each individual situation needs to be looked at by the co-ordinator of volunteers and appropriate other staff members before a decision is made.

A volunteer needs to be physically and emotionally ready to work with people who are dying. There is no person with greater empathy for a patient than one with experience of illness but only when that person is ready.

The palliative care volunteer is given a copy of the mission statement, policies, aims, procedures, guidelines (see the Appendix), and job description of a palliative care volunteer at the beginning of the initial education programme.

A statement of commitment, promising to work for at least 12 months, is signed by the volunteer before beginning work in the hospital.

Areas where volunteers do not work

There are some areas in the work of the palliative care service where volunteers are never put.

Included in these is when a patient has a 'nuclear hazard' sign on the door of his/her room. The volunteer then would not visit that patient for 48–72 hours after treatment, whilst radiation remains active. Another example is if a patient has a 'do not disturb' sign on his/her door, when the volunteer is asked to check with the nursing staff to see if this includes volunteers. Often, this sign is only meant for visitors.

Volunteer work areas

Day roster

On day roster the volunteers work in the two wards and day care oncology. They spend one day a week for a month in each place. It is important that the patients get to know the volunteers when in the acute care part of the hospital as this means that they already feel comfortable with them when they subsequently meet them in the palliative care unit.

Haematology/oncology wards

If the volunteers are in the haematology/oncology wards or day care oncology they need to check which patients are 'palliative care patients'. They have priority but the volunteers also visit the other patients in these areas.

On each haematology/oncology ward the volunteers visit the patients offering to do anything they can for the patient within the volunteer guidelines (see the Appendix). Quite often, it is simply to have a talk to fill the patient's time. Sometimes, these talks can disclose information that needs to be passed on to a staff member. On such occasions the volunteer will encourage the patient to speak to a specific staff member.

Volunteers also help with grooming and/or helping the patient to manage his/her food. The volunteer may encourage or help the patient to write his/her memoirs or read to the patient. If a patient is very unwell, the relative or friend who visits the patient regularly often appreciates the company of a volunteer.

Day oncology

In day oncology, where patients have chemotherapy or other day procedures, volunteers have a short chat with the patient and often with a family member or friend who is accompanying the patient. They make a cup of tea or coffee for the patients and distribute the lunches. There is a fairly rapid turnover of patients so the volunteers are kept busy.

Palliative care unit

Volunteers do similar work in both the cancer wards and the palliative care unit. Here, they spend more time sitting holding a patient's hand and helping with meals. They also take the patients for a ride in a wheelchair around the hospital grounds. This brings the patient into contact with the world outside and gives him/her an opportunity to smell the flowers and feel the sun, etc. Volunteers also sit with dying patients if they have no family or friends present at this time.

Another volunteer occupation in this unit is spending time with patients' families either beside the patient's bed or in the lounge rooms. In this unit the volunteers take around the drinks trolley at lunch time.

Radiotherapy unit

Volunteers visit the radiotherapy waiting rooms and spend time waiting with the patients. This gives both the patient and their carer another chance to get to know the volunteers. It also gives the volunteer an opportunity perhaps to discover a patient's need while the patient is still staying at home.

Evening roster

This is between 16:00 and 18:00 hours with two different volunteers on duty in each area.

The evening roster begins with a drink round where the volunteer takes a trolley of both soft drinks and alcohol to the patient's bedside or, if the patients are mobile, to a sitting room for pre-dinner drinks. (No alcohol is ever given to a visitor.) When this round is completed the volunteer is then available to assist patients who need help with eating their meals.

The main point to emphasize is that volunteers help only when the patients cannot do things for themselves. Patients need to retain as much independence as possible.

This evening roster is usually a very pleasant, relaxed time for both volunteers and patients. Often, volunteers who cannot help during the day because of other commitments are able to help at this time.

'One-to-one'

A volunteer who works with a particular patient on a regular basis is called a 'one-to-one' or '1/1' volunteer. This really symbolizes how a 1/1 volunteer stands beside a patient with a connecting link between them.

Such 1/1 volunteers are usually allocated to patients with extra needs such as those:

(1) from the country, some distance from the hospital;

(2) with very few or even no visitors;

(3) who are going to be in the hospital a long time;

(4) who need extra emotional support;

(5) whose relatives or friends doing most of the caring need extra support.

This 1/1 volunteer will visit this particular patient regularly, perhaps two or three times a week while in hospital and will take a special interest in this patient each time he/she comes to the hospital either for outpatient, radiotherapy or day oncology visits.

The patient/volunteer 'match' must always be kept in mind when selecting a 1/1 volunteer. The patient always has the right to refuse a visit from a volunteer. Volunteers are selected for this volunteer role according to the needs of the patients. This means that volunteers, even if they are able to do so, may not always have a 1/1 patient.

It is hoped that one day there will be sufficient volunteers to be able to assign *each* patient a 1/1 volunteer when they are given palliative care status.

Special work

Many volunteers have special talents, which they bring to the hospital such as painting, meditation, massage, hairdressing or craft, etc. If it is appropriate and in accordance with the hospital's policy, such volunteers are invited to use these talents for groups or individual patients. Others volunteer with valuable previous experience (e.g. in fund-raising) in which case they would be placed in that department (see below).

Office work

There are volunteers who, for many different reasons, prefer to work in the office rather than with the patients so they are trained to organize the rosters, write the newsletter, keep the statistics up to date, and many other ongoing tasks.

Fund-raising

The fund-raising team has one or two fund-raising efforts each year. This money is used to buy drinks for the drink trolleys, for volunteer education and further training courses, as well as to buy specific items of equipment for the palliative care service such as an oxygen concentrator.

♦ There is a fund-raising and volunteers office in our hospital and this department's manager is the person responsible for both fund-raising and volunteer services. There is also a manager of volunteers in this office who is responsible for all other managers of volunteers in the hospital. The Palliative Care Volunteer Services Manager (PCVSM) registers the palliative care volunteers with this manager of volunteers. This department covers all volunteers for insurance.

This manager of volunteers must be notified, usually verbally, of any activities affecting the hospital or advertised outside the hospital including fund-raising (e.g. when education programmes are scheduled and advertised).

♦ The fund-raising for the hospital is organized by a volunteer committee with many auxiliaries throughout the suburbs who work closely with the manager of the fund-raising and volunteers office. There are other co-ordinators for volunteer driving of patients to appointments, the canteen and coffee shops, the accident and emergency volunteers, the volunteers in other wards. All co-ordinators of volunteers are under the umbrella of this central department but answer to our own departments first.

♦ In the palliative care volunteer service, the group of palliative care fund-raising volunteers would report to the PCVSM informally then report formally at the palliative care volunteers' monthly meeting where the decision to go ahead with a specific fund-raising venture would be decided. The palliative care volunteer service would then ask permission for this activity from the manager of the fund-raising and volunteers office in a formal letter.

At the end of a roster

When volunteers are finished for the day they return to the office, fill in the report forms, write patient notes, and sign off before saying goodbye to the VSM. If the volunteer is going to be absent at any time he/she makes a note in the holiday book so that when the rosters are being prepared for the next month these dates can be taken into consideration.

Regular ongoing training and education of volunteers

One of our aims, as Volunteer Service Managers working in palliative care, should be to educate the volunteers to be professional palliative care volunteers.

Professional means '(a) having or showing the skill of a professional, competent; (b) worthy of a professional (professional conduct)'.[1]

In the palliative care volunteer service being described there is an initial education programme followed by further educational opportunities to enhance skills and knowledge by such means as monthly meetings, training as mentors, the advanced palliative care workers education programme, and external education courses each year.

Initial pre-service training

It is very important to carefully select and train the palliative care volunteers *before* they begin working with the patients.

Experience shows that it is better to have *fewer* but good quality volunteers than *more* volunteers who, for one reason or another, turn out to be unsuitable.

Subjects covered in our *40 hours initial training programme* include:

- palliative care—philosophy and practice;
- confidentiality;
- rights and responsibilities of volunteers;
- rights and responsibilities of patients;
- spirituality;
- ethical issues;
- culture and religion;
- sexuality and illness;
- the vulnerability of being a patient;
- death, grief and loss.

The volunteer also needs to know and be comfortable with him/herself before he/she can be comfortable with a patient who is dying.

The most important part of the programme is communication so 20 hours of the programme is devoted to this subject. It is essential for a volunteer to be able to listen and to communicate extremely well with a patient.

Occupational therapy, physiotherapy, and diet in palliative care are discussed by the palliative care team with the student volunteers. Radiotherapy and chemotherapy are also mentioned.

When the volunteers finish the programme they are *again* interviewed. If they are suitable they then begin working in the hospital with a mentor.

Monthly in-service training

There are regular monthly meetings for volunteers with one hour allocated to education and one hour for debriefing and general discussion. Prior to the meeting a newsletter including minutes of the previous meeting and rosters for the next month are sent to each volunteer.

The volunteers share lunch before this meeting. A speaker is invited to address a list of queries about palliative care which volunteers prepared at the beginning of the year.

If there is a patient with an illness or a specific problem that the volunteers need more education about, then the VSM would ask the appropriate staff member to speak instead of someone from the list of speakers.

External education

The volunteers are encouraged to attend palliative care or volunteer education programmes offered by other organizations. The costs of attending these are often subsidized by the service.

Advanced education for palliative care workers

It was found that the volunteers had many questions and wanted more education after they had been working with patients for a few months. A survey was conducted asking what information and further training were wanted. This resulted in the 20 hours advanced palliative care workers' education programme being offered each year. To qualify for it participants must have worked in palliative care for at least six months before undertaking this study.

In the *20 hours advanced training programme* we take time to go more deeply into subjects such as:

+ radiotherapy;
+ chemotherapy;
+ the cell cycle and cancer;
+ grief;
+ bereavement;
+ complementary therapies;
+ cancer research;
+ dying in a palliative care unit;
+ dying at home; and
+ other subjects to help the volunteers' understanding of palliative care in the home and in hospital.

The assessments after each course have shown that the programme is well received by both palliative care and pastoral care volunteers working in palliative care from around the state.

Mentors

A 'mentor' is a person who has been a palliative care volunteer for at least 12 months and is considered suitable to mentor or guide another volunteer. Not all volunteers wish to be a mentor and certainly being a good volunteer him/herself does not necessarily make him/her a good mentor. These volunteers then participate in a four to six hour mentor training course which includes how to:

- communicate by discussing or offering suggestions in a positive way;
- support and encourage the new volunteer;
- report to the VSM verbally (informally) and written (formally) on the progress of the new volunteer;
- show new volunteers where to locate people and places;
- help the new volunteer to fill in forms, and deal with documentation.

The role of the VSM in the debriefing of volunteers

There are several opportunities for debriefing:

1 When a patient dies there is a debriefing of staff on the ward and volunteers are encouraged to go to these sessions, which are usually organized by the nurse unit manager (sister in charge of the ward) or a palliative care staff member.

2 At the volunteers' monthly meetings we also talk about the patients' deaths and any issues that the volunteers raise.

3 Once or twice a year, or when there is a need, someone is asked to come in and debrief the group or speak about looking after oneself.

4 It is also very important for the VSM to formally debrief on a regular basis as well as having someone for the volunteer to talk to at any time.

5 If a volunteer has been a 1/1 with a patient who dies or has been particularly close to a patient in the unit I always notify them of that patient's death and chat to them about how they feel.

6 If it is felt anyone needs a special debriefing then that will be done. Either the VSM will debrief the volunteer or if more appropriate, will get one of the staff, such as the social worker or the pastoral care person from the palliative care service, to meet with him/her.

'Burn-out'

It is important to be conscious of the possibility of volunteer burn-out. This is why it is so important for the VSM to be readily available to drop everything and spend time with the volunteer if that is needed.

My policy has been to have an open door and I find this works much better than having only specific report/debriefing times. By this I mean that I encourage the volunteers to greet me when they arrive and to again call by my office as they leave. During this time we usually chat about how their day went in a very informal way and I can usually pick up if there is something that is worrying them or that they feel needs to be looked into for a patient. Then, if necessary, we talk more seriously about this either then or at an appointed time. Sometimes, it is something I have to take up with someone else and then I let the volunteer know the results of the follow-up.

If a volunteer seems to be tired all the time or irritable or just seems uninterested in everything, this could be a sign he/she is exhausted mentally or physically. I discuss with the volunteer if it is to do with his/her work with palliative care or if it is from something going on in his/her life outside the hospital.

If it is something that is more serious or is something from his/her life outside we sometimes agree that it would be wise for the volunteer to have some time off. We set a specific length to this time (e.g. two weeks, three months), or what seems appropriate, then review this at a later date. During this time off duty I maintain contact with the volunteer by telephone.

Another option is to have the volunteers work for a short time in the office or elsewhere where there is no patient contact.

Many volunteers need to move on after a few years working in palliative care either because they need a change or because of changed circumstances in their life. It is important to recognize and to acknowledge the work they have done for the patients and the palliative care service

Burn-out is something that the VSM must watch for in him/herself. It is helpful to make a list of your favourite things that you can use to help relax you on a regular basis. Time away from one's regular routine is also beneficial.

Delegating responsibility

The primary duty of the VSM is to '*be there*' for the volunteers, to be readily available. By delegating tasks this allows the VSM to be available rather than getting bogged down in routine office work

Organizing and ordering supplies is one task that can be delegated as can setting up rooms for meetings, minute taking, and writing reports on meetings. The formation of a volunteer fund-raising committee could also be delegated.

When it is planned to delegate responsibility to someone or to start something new, it is always discussed at the regular meetings of volunteers, clear plans drawn up and a 'job description' prepared for whoever is asked to take on the responsibility. Reports from the person taking on the role are then presented at the regular volunteer meetings.

It is important that the VSM always knows what is going on by showing an interest without seeming to check-up or override the volunteers' decisions. Regular written reports from the delegated volunteers are important. Duties should be interesting and fulfilling to the delegated volunteer.

Accountability of the VSM

In the hospital on which this chapter has been based, the VSM answers to the nurse consultant co-ordinator of palliative care services first, but also to the manager of volunteers for the whole hospital.

Selecting volunteers for specific work

Volunteers who look after the specific parts of the programme are those who:

+ have a special interest in that area;

+ have already shown a talent in that specific area;

+ offered themselves as volunteers knowing they had a particular skill or experience that might be useful.

Most volunteers come having heard of the work 'by word of mouth' but a few respond to advertisements. In that case, whatever special qualities they may have are discussed with them. They are asked if they have had the experience of having someone close to them die. It is possible from an initial informal chat that enough information is provided to decide whether to give them an application form or to advise them against applying. The application form asks among other things for special qualities, gifts or skills. If these skills are appropriate the prospective volunteers are asked if they would be willing to use their talent with the patients. (We do not have children under the age of 16 in the cancer wards because they go to the children's hospital.)

Sometimes, volunteers are voted in at a meeting while at other times I personally invite them to undertake a task. Asking people to take responsibility for something that they are good at is a way of showing that what they do is noticed and appreciated.

It is very important to thank volunteers for what they do for the patients, the staff, and especially for helping the VSM.

When problems arise

If, on the other hand, a problem arises with a volunteer the VSM will need to discuss the issue with him/her as soon as possible. It is always important to be honest with a volunteer but discuss the problem gently with him/her rather than say 'you are wrong'.

Quite often you will find that they too are not happy with what is going on but do not know what to do to change things. An open discussion allowing the volunteer to express his/her feelings, then working on the problem together and if possible getting them to find a solution makes things easier for everyone. In fact, this usually strengthens the volunteer's commitment to the palliative care service and to yourself as his/her VSM.

It is important for a volunteer to know that you respect his/her confidentiality just as you expect him/her to respect the confidentiality of patients and staff.

If the problem is between two volunteers, the VSM usually talks to them separately then if they cannot solve the problem themselves the VSM meets with them together and oversees the discussion. Sometimes, the circumstances are too raw and another action has to be taken (perhaps by transferring one or both to another duty). If it is not a major problem affecting the hospital or patients then it is sometimes better to let things rest for a while before instigating a meeting. This gives them time to cool down and think things through.

Key point: Remember, the patient's comfort is of the utmost importance.

When having a discussion with the volunteers about a problem I bring questions like these into the conversation:

+ 'Why are you here?'

+ 'Who have you come here to help?'

+ 'Is this situation helping either the patient or you?'

+ 'Is this too stressful for you or are you bringing your personal life into your voluntary work?'

+ 'Do you need time off?'

For *major* problems with both staff and volunteers there is a laid down hospital procedure. If a volunteer has to be asked to leave it can usually be done by discussion and mutual agreement.

Aiming for a more comprehensive palliative care service

What could make a good palliative care volunteer service an even better one? What follow are my personal views, based on many years experience.

1 The structures to set up and run extra programmes take time that is not available with only a part-time VSM therefore a *full-time VSM and a part-time assistant* would be an asset. This would allow the VSM more time for specialized volunteer training therefore preparing the volunteers to do more for the patients.

2 It is important for the volunteers to be able to speak to someone whenever they need to. If the VSM is not available then someone, preferably the assistant VSM, or another nominated member of the palliative care team should be available.

3 To be able to give each patient a one-to-one volunteer as soon as his/her diagnosis is palliative would be ideal. This volunteer can be there for them through all his/her visits to the hospital—this would necessitate many more volunteers.

4 Three shifts a day on all cancer wards especially the palliative care unit are desirable. A morning roster from say 07:00 to 09:00 hours would enable volunteers to help patients with their self-care if need be and also with breakfast while the nurses are at the busiest time of their shift. If patients can have their personal care (shave, hair set, nails clipped, and painted, etc.) completed early in the day it helps them to face another day more confidently.

The volunteer only does what the patient needs and wants. This leaves the patient with as much independence as possible, for example, the patient may be able to shave himself quite well but cannot reach the razor in the drawer. *Note*: volunteers should never overwhelm patients.

The relationship between volunteers and staff

There is an agreement between the union and the manager of all the hospital volunteers as to how many hours a volunteer may work in a week. It is important to ensure that no volunteer works more than this number of hours or you will jeopardize the programme. In this hospital, this agreement is for 16 hours per week per volunteer.

Another important policy of the hospital is that volunteers may not do any of the work of paid staff. That is to say, they complement but never replace paid staff. This applies even when a health care professional offers his/her services as a volunteer. If they are placed in a clinical environment they report to whoever is in charge of that unit of the hospital but do not replace any salaried member of staff. Never having had a doctor volunteer it is not possible to say what would be the case there.

It is wise for the manager of palliative care volunteers to regularly speak to staff individually or in groups about the volunteers' work.

Annual review

There is an annual review of each palliative care volunteer which includes a written questionnaire and an interview. At this interview we set the aims the volunteer has for the next 12 months as a palliative care volunteer as well as discussing the questionnaire and any other issues. Even though these interviews take many hours I find that they are well worth the time spent.

Conclusion

The co-ordinator (as we still call her) or Voluntary Service Manager, must always consider him/herself first—remembering that he/she is not there to solve all the problems of the patients or volunteers. It is vitally important to ensure that there is someone who has time to debrief the VSM regularly and that the VSM has other interests in order to relax.

Regular meetings with the multidisciplinary palliative care service in the hospital are essential as these meetings keep the professional palliative care team up to date with what is happening in the volunteer team, and the volunteer team with what is happening in the hospital. It is the responsibility of the VSM to update the team on volunteer activities.

It raises the profile of the volunteer team if the VSM takes a volunteer on a rotating basis to such meetings, discussing ideas in advance with the volunteer to save embarrassment.

Regular, even frequent, meetings with other co-ordinators of palliative care volunteers/VSMs in the city or district, can be very useful—sharing information and ideas, collaborating in education and training courses, being mutually supportive. It can be so helpful and reassuring to find that many problems and challenges are common to them all.

Appendix
Austin & Repatriation Medical Service, Palliative Care Volunteer Service
Guidelines for volunteers*

1. Three months after a volunteer accepts his/her first patient or begins on the wards, there shall be a confidential review with the co-ordinator of the volunteer's role, thereafter an annual review will occur.

2. Observe confidentiality of patient, staff and volunteers at all times.

3. In an emergency situation call the nurse immediately.

4. Don't comment on a patient's treatment or medical condition.

5. Don't offer advice regarding a patient's personal or family matters. Generally, you can best help the patient or caregiver by letting them talk about their problems and by being a good listener.

6. Respect the right to privacy of patients and their relations.

7. Leave your own attitudes, values and problems behind when you visit patients and their families. Treat the patient and family with the respect they deserve as fellow human beings.

8. Recognize and refer when a problem is beyond your abilities or your volunteer role. Inform the Co-ordinator of Volunteers or other Palliative Care Staff when problem situations arise or when professional or specialist intervention should be sought.

9. It is important that you care for yourself. There are times when your own emotional needs may have to come first. Don't be afraid to say 'No' if you are uncomfortable with a person or a situation. Try not to take problems away with you and recognize your own limitations.

10. Don't comment to patients on other patients or staff members.

11. Money and gifts are not to be accepted by volunteers. If a patient or relative wishes to make a personal gift, advise them that donations may be made to the Palliative Care Volunteer Service.

12. Do NOT give out your telephone number or address. Patients and caregivers can contact you through the Co-ordinator of Palliative Care Volunteers.

13. While how you dress may not matter to some patients, that may not always be the case. Be neat and appropriately dressed when visiting patients and their families.

14. A written report is required at the end of each day's activities.

15. Report regularly to the Co-ordinator of Palliative Care Volunteers. This will provide the support you need and keep the team informed so that the patient receives optimal care.

*Reproduced with permission from the Austin & Repatriation Medical Service, Melbourne, Victoria, Australia.

Reference

Moore B (ed.) (1997). *The Australian concise Oxford Dictionary of current english,* (3rd edn). Oxford University Press, Melbourne, Australia.

Recommended reading

Jordan L and Hanley R (2001). *Guidelines for volunteers.* Palliative Care Volunteer Service, Austin & Repatriation Medical Centre, Melbourne, Victoria, Australia.

Chapter 8

Volunteers working in a community palliative care service

Dame Cicely Saunders brought the hospice concept to South Africa in 1979. The traditional British model was introduced by various groups of volunteers across the country during the early 1980s. This chapter describes how volunteers work in what might be regarded by many in the developed world as an unusual, even a unique, community palliative care service in South Africa.

South Coast Hospice, Kwazulu-Natal, South Africa

South Coast Hospice (SCH) is situated on the eastern seaboard of South Africa alongside the Indian Ocean on the southern coast of Kwazulu-Natal. It serves the UGU South Health District* that extends over approximately 3385 square kilometres and has its headquarters in the town of Port Shepstone, just over an hour's drive south of Durban. (See Figures 8.1 and 8.2.)

In the absence of accurate figures, the population is *estimated* to be in excess of 650 000. Unemployment in this impoverished area is >70%.[1] The prevalence of tuberculosis is one of the highest in the world, and was already 116 per 100 000 in 1998.[2] A survey by Murchison Hospital which serves the area indicated that 82% of people with TB are also HIV positives.[3] It is further estimated that in South Africa as a whole 4.7 million people have HIV/AIDS, one of the highest rates in the world.

The people of the area served by South Coast Hospice and its community palliative care service have access to primary care clinics offering round-the-clock cost-free care. In addition there are small hospitals offering 24 hour care, with minimal charges for medications. The clinics and the hospitals are state-run and state-funded unlike the palliative care services.

General practitioners (GPs) are readily accessible in urban areas. Patients may choose which ones to consult but must pay fees, which usually include medications, usually much higher than a hospital would charge. Medications are usually purchased at a local pharmacy.

* UGU is a Zulu word meaning 'the coast'.

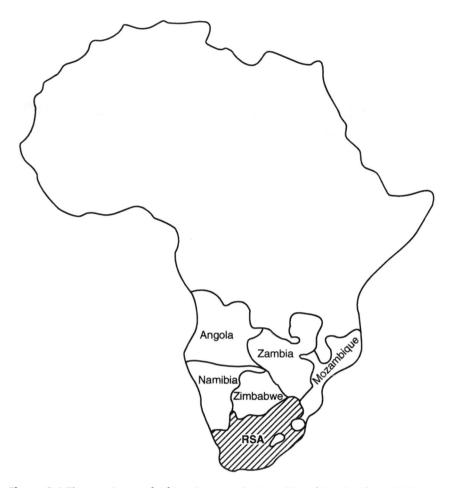

Figure 8.1 The continent of Africa showing the Republic of South Africa (RSA).

The impact of HIV/AIDS

The magnitude of the HIV/AIDS problem has already been alluded to. The problems faced by the patients and carers are more than physical. The psychological effects and the stigma related to HIV vary as the infection progresses.

At the initial 'well-but-worried' and healthy carrier stage, adequate counselling is often not sought. The infected person tries to come to terms with his/her diagnosis and goes through a series of psychological reactions, shock, fear, denial, anger, blame, and guilt. These universal reactions seem to be exacerbated in the case of a person living with HIV/AIDS (usually abbreviated to PWA). There is often a high level of stigma and lack of acceptance of the PWA. People are frightened or ashamed of having a PWA in their home. This makes it difficult for a volunteer/caregiver to have access at this time. It often takes a while for these people to disclose their status to the family.

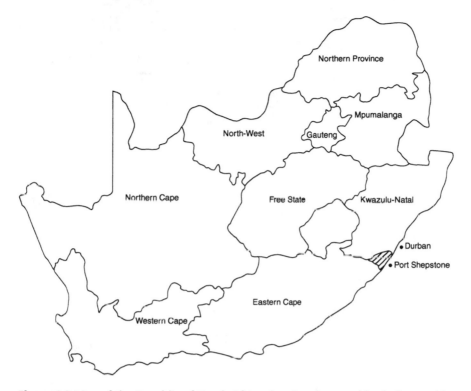

Figure 8.2 Map of the Republic of South Africa showing the area (shaded) served by the South Coast Hospice.

The bulk of the volunteer involvement about to be described occurs when the PWA is already ill. As a result the volunteer frequently has to deal not only with the terminally ill patient but also an overwhelmed family and the problem of stigma.

In excess of 60% of PWAs referred to South Coast Hospice (SCH) are female. More than 80% of all infected women acquire HIV infection from a male partner to whom they have been faithful.[5] It takes a very competent volunteer to talk openly about sexuality and related health problems in a culture where such discussion is taboo. 'Vulnerability to AIDS is often associated with a lack of respect for the rights of women and children'.[6] The problem is exacerbated when the volunteer is young and/or unmarried and has to deal with an older male who is culturally perceived as powerful. A relationship of trust is crucial for effective ongoing counselling and care to occur.

Figure 8.3 and Table 8.1 are taken from the UGU South HIV/AIDS/STD/TB Pilot Site Interim Report covering the period October 1999 to April 2001. This SCH research project verified the magnitude of the impact of HIV/AIDS in their operational area of rural Kwazulu-Natal.[7]

In view of the fact that anti-retroviral medications are at the time of writing not available in South Africa, virtually *all* these HIV positive people will be requiring

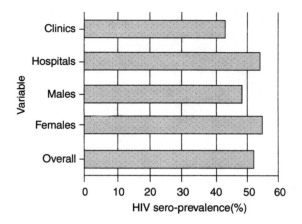

Figure 8.3 HIV sero-prevalence of 12 000 clients tested at Port Shepstone regional Hospital (Data collected September 1998–November 1999).

Table 8.1 Five main reasons given for a self-referral for HIV/AIDS (April 1998–May 2000)

Reason for self-referral	Number (%)
1. Interested after health education talk	1801 (73%)
2. Client is ill	357 (14%)
3. Client concerned about his/her risk activities	037 (12%)
4. Client concerned about partner's risk activities	149 (6%)
5. Partner is ill or has died	51 (2%)

palliative care within the near future. Clearly, the need for dedicated volunteers will therefore escalate considerably.

The history of volunteer involvement

South Coast Hospice has been forced to develop innovative ways of coping with the overwhelming and escalating number of HIV positive people in their region who are in desperate need of holistic palliative care. How this has been done is the subject of this chapter.

The area served by the SCH is not affluent, the only two large commercial ventures being a cement factory and sugar mill. Most jobs are associated with agriculture or tourism. SCH is severely restricted by financial constraints, support from the government is very limited and only accounted for 6% of the 2001 annual budget. All these factors resulted in SCH focusing on training *lay* community caregivers and volunteers to do work that is traditionally done by nurses and social workers. Professional nurses and social workers have in turn been required to concentrate on supporting and supervising these lay caregivers. The challenge of providing quality of care in this context is never lost sight of.

As early as 1984, SCH found it necessary to adapt the British model and began collaborating with primary health care clinics in order to provide holistic care to

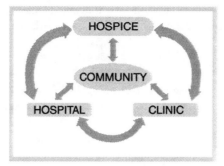

Figure 8.4 Integrated community-based home care (ICHC).

cancer patients living in the outlying rural areas. Many of the professional nurses who were working in outlying primary health care clinics became hospice volunteers. Now, most volunteers are not trained nurses but lay women eager to help people in their own district, usually within walking distance of their own home. Working in this way in their own community means that the volunteers are well known and relatively safe, although they are advised to work with a partner for additional support.

This rural outreach programme laid the foundation for the integrated community-based home care (ICHC) model that came about in 1996, in response to the escalating HIV/AIDS epidemic (see Figure 8.4). SCH is currently associated with 24 permanent clinics as well as the mobile clinic network. As indicated above and in Fig. 8.3, the problem of AIDS, and AIDS orphans in particular is huge. SCH statistics show an average of 3.6 potential orphans per household. At the end of October 2001 there were 477 households with HIV positive patients on the ICHC programme.

Definition of a volunteer

Volunteers form an integral and enriching part of hospices all over the world. To volunteer is to give service willingly of one's own accord. The biblical adage that in giving we receive, is true. The satisfaction that comes from making a positive difference in difficult circumstances is definitely rewarding.

In the developed world it goes without saying that no monetary payment is expected, or received, when one volunteers. However, this may not be the case when people from an impoverished background 'volunteer'. Their motivation may well be two-fold. They genuinely wish to be of service and simultaneously hope that this 'volunteering' will lead to a job or gain them some incentive that will help alleviate their own plight by assisting them to feed themselves and their family. In view of this the concept of a 'paid volunteer' is therefore not as strange as it may first seem. Individual hospices in Kwazulu-Natal are currently grappling with sustainable ways of addressing this problem.

Volunteer rewards range from food parcels to financial stipends equal to a nominal salary. The number of volunteers, their commitment and the approximate number of hours they devote to the hospice are some of the factors that need to be considered. To prevent conflict it is important to have a clear policy that is strictly adhered to and communicated to all concerned.

Selection of volunteers

Careful selection becomes even more important when payment of volunteers may be involved. It is therefore vital to ascertain the true motivation of any potential volunteer.

The universal qualities required for a person who will be working as a volunteer member of a team anywhere include:

- personal warmth;
- a non-judgemental attitude to those with HIV/AIDS;
- ability to communicate effectively;
- respectful and positive attitude to HIV status;
- flexibility and emotional maturity;
- well balanced lifestyle;
- good coping mechanisms.

In South Africa *additional* characteristics found to be important include:

- a track record of community involvement;
- the ability to communicate cross-culturally with sensitivity and respect;
- the ability to converse in a knowledgeable and compassionate manner about HIV/AIDS.

Almost all volunteers are women because, traditionally and culturally, the women are the carers in this society. Caring is seen as one of their responsibilities.

There is a surprisingly low turnover of community-based volunteers. The most common reason for resignation is that they have secured a better paid position. When this occurs the hospice celebrates with them and they continue to be valuable ambassadors for the organization. Even when volunteers leave the geographical area they frequently volunteer for similar work in their new place of residence.

Introducing volunteers to the work

As important pillars in the provision of care it is necessary for volunteers, not only to be adequately trained for the work but also to be introduced to the key figures and all relevant role players in the community they will be serving. These include representatives from various government departments, non-governmental community-based-organizations and recognized community leaders. At the same time, the community needs to be informed about the programme as well as the role of the volunteer. Scheduled community meetings can often be used for this purpose.

It is also necessary to orientate all hospice professional staff regarding the training, skills and areas of volunteer operation. In addition to making the volunteer feel a part of the organization, importantly, proper orientation also enhances the referral system.

The new volunteer needs to be given information about the correct channels of communication. They need to understand about supervision and relevant networking resources, in keeping with their specific job description. To avoid tensions building up between lay volunteers and hospice professionals working relationships must be clearly defined from the outset. It is also important they be made aware of the need for flexibility. SCH volunteers are rotated through the in-patient unit and must, of necessity, be prepared to work in a variety of areas. Experienced volunteers are often expected to shoulder additional responsibilities and mentor new recruits.

Relationship of volunteers to professionals

Whenever volunteers are involved in giving direct patient care it is necessary to stress professional accountability. It is essential to have clear job descriptions that set out what is expected of the volunteer and also what he/she is not permitted to do.

As a general rule, non-professional volunteers and all lay caregivers do not liaise *directly* with professionals from other organizations. If volunteers encounter a problem when visiting a patient they have access to registered nurses based at the primary health care clinics scattered across the country. These nurses provide interim professional support until the problem can be reported to a palliative care nurse at the base palliative care unit/hospice. Should medical help be needed it is the palliative care *nurse*, not the volunteer, who brings the matter to the doctor's attention.

Volunteers may only administer medication according to a strict protocol. Generally speaking, they do not do so but they are permitted to help a patient or relative to measure medicines. They do not carry out any invasive procedures.

The Hospice Association of South Africa (HASA) has adopted and piloted the ICHC model (see Figure 8.4) in which hospices also work closely with various other HIV/AIDS community-based initiatives. The HIV/AIDS epidemic has motivated numerous South African hospices to implement this practical model of care.

How integrated home-based home care operates

People living with HIV/AIDS (PWA) are identified at local hospitals and visited by South Coast Hospice community caregivers. The team transport patients home on discharge and inform the relevant primary health care clinic. A full patient/family assessment is carried out and a care plan compiled on the first home visit.

Hospice care teams (salaried professional staff) visit on average once a week, interim support and care being provided by the trained lay volunteers who live within walking distance of the patients' homes.

On average, each lay volunteer has about five patients and their families to visit. At the end of each week each volunteer meets with the Voluntary Service Manager (VSM) and the nurses and reports on the week's work.

In the event of problems developing between the weekly visits, volunteers and/or family members consult with a professional nurse at the clinic who will give advice and medication if appropriate or, in the case of an emergency, arrange for admission to hospital. Hospice caregivers and volunteers network with various other role players such as churches, women's groups, traditional healers and other relevant individuals and groups, to obtain additional support for patients and their families. The core elements of the ICHC model (see also Figure 8.4) include:

◆ linking palliative home-based care to preventive care;

◆ providing a continuum of care;

◆ drawing on the strengths already existing in community-based care initiatives;

◆ integrating the statutory and private health care sectors;

◆ training people from the community as caregivers and providing them with jobs;

◆ enhancing the morale of *all* health care providers;

◆ capitalizing on important teaching opportunities;

◆ using volunteers to complement a small core of salaried community caregivers

All care is audited on a six monthly basis, using an audit tool developed by the Hospice Association of South Africa (HASA) (see Appendices 1–3) during the piloting of the ICHC model.

Although paid community caregivers are crucially important to the ICHC model, lay volunteers have played a pivotal role in its success. The small core of paid caregivers can only manage to visit patients once a week, all others being done by the lay volunteers. In addition to the current four ICHC teams that each cover a specific geographical area, there is a specialized children's team—so great is the problem of children with HIV/AIDS.

The work of volunteers

In South Coast Hospice, as in many hospices, the traditional roles for volunteers include:

◆ Direct patient and family care.

◆ Fund-raising.

◆ Administration.

◆ Financial management.

◆ Numerous support and consultancy services.

In keeping with the holistic care requirements of the developing world, hospices in Kwazulu-Natal also use volunteers for:

◆ Community development.

◆ Poverty alleviation.

◆ Orphan care.

◆ HIV/AIDS awareness and prevention programmes.

All this has become necessary because the traditional safety net provided by the extended family system in rural African communities is being eroded by HIV/AIDS.[4] In addition, there are the continuing social problems of poverty, unemployment, and domestic violence.[4] Over-burdened grandmothers, who are themselves in need of bereavement support, cannot possibly cope with caring for their own sick children and grandchildren as well as inheriting the orphans. According to SCH statistics, 40% of orphaned children are themselves HIV positive. This places an unimaginable burden on these elderly women, often themselves ill and frail and underfed.

Training

Ideally, volunteers should receive initial training:

- in their own geographical area;
- in an environment with which they are familiar;
- preferably in their own language.

Familiarizing them with community resources and how to access them forms part of this initial training. Training is based on the three month Hospice Association of South Africa (HASA) curriculum. When circumstances do not permit for the entire curriculum to be completed initially, core elements of each of the modules are incorporated into a one month course and the balance incorporated into ongoing/inservice training.

The curriculum is divided into the following eight modules and learning outcomes:

1 Introductory module—HIV/AIDS in context

On completion of this module the volunteer must be able to demonstrate an understanding of the basic facts regarding the mode of transmission, prevention, and factors increasing the risk of the spread of HIV/AIDS and the role of home-based care.

2 The community caregiver

This includes an assessment by the student of his/her own values and attitudes to HIV/AIDS, as well as community misconceptions and myths. The role of the caregiver, rules of conduct, ethical principles, and professional approach, as well as support systems available to the caregiver.

3 Basic communication skills

On completion of this module the volunteer is expected to be able to demonstrate effective communication skills and the use of interpersonal skills to establish rapport with patients and families, use correct referral procedures, keep accurate records, and have an awareness of ethical and legal issues.

4 Psychosocial and spiritual support

The social, emotional, and spiritual impact of the disease on the individual and family; the dying process; loss, grief, and bereavement, and how to offer support are covered in this module.

5 Basic nursing skills—including the philosophy of holistic care

Volunteers must be able to maintain basic hygiene and apply universal precautions in preventing the spread of infection, demonstrate a basic understanding of all the body systems, recognize specific problems related to HIV/AIDS, and be able to utilize this knowledge in the appropriate care of patients. They also need to be able to give sound nutritional guidance to patients and families.

6 Pain and symptom control

In terms of learning outcomes the volunteer must be able to demonstrate an understanding of total pain and its effect on the patient; identify non-pharmaceutical methods of pain relief and utilize simple appropriate measures for relieving pain. They must also work under professional supervision in the administration of prescribed medication. Students must be able to give an accurate report on all aspects of the patient's condition and employ proper storage and record keeping of medicines.

7 Paediatric AIDS

This module deals with all aspects of the disease and treatment related specifically to children. The volunteers are required to identify and respond to specific HIV/AIDS problems that relate to infants, children, and teenagers.

8 Teaching methods module

This is included so that community caregivers and volunteers are able to use relevant teaching methods to convey information to patients, families and communities, and use knowledge to empower their own communities in self-help.

Once the three month basic training is completed, volunteers are encouraged in identifying their own ongoing training needs. Volunteers bring with them a wide range of valuable experience that can often be appropriately channelled into peer training.

Support

Training forms an important part of volunteer support in that it affirms their competency and contributes to their personal development and confidence. Community recognition of the sacrifice and committed dedication of volunteers is of paramount importance and certainly contributes to their sustainability.

Personal supervision and mentorship

Volunteers, particularly those working in impoverished and traumatic conditions need to be able to vent their feelings and talk about how the work is affecting them personally. Time needs to be scheduled for volunteers to have regular sessions with a suitably skilled psychosocial professional individually and/or in groups. In order to avoid 'burn-out', volunteers are encouraged to set limits and work within a scheduled time-frame. They are also encouraged to take time off on a regular basis.

Recognition

A badge or uniform means a great deal to hospice volunteers who are proud to be associated with the organization. Thanking volunteers encourages and motivates them, particularly when this is done in public. It makes profound sense to ensure that the contribution made by volunteers is stressed in all relevant reports. Everyone likes to be appreciated.

Volunteers associated with Kwazulu-Natal hospices together with their partners, are invited to attend two annual events—a 'Thanksgiving and Remembrance service' and a Christmas party.

Monitoring and evaluation

It is as important to monitor the quality of work done by volunteers as that done by salaried staff. With adequate preparation and a non-threatening approach this can be perceived as uplifting and give volunteers a feeling of security. Regular assessment and feedback regarding the quality of their work is another way of telling volunteers that they are important.

Having a policy regarding the monitoring and evaluation of volunteers in place makes it easier to respond effectively to incidences of misconduct. For instance, the breaking of patient confidentiality is regarded as a dismissable offence. Evaluating the quality of work simultaneously monitors the effectiveness and relevance of existing training programmes. It also highlights areas that need to be included in ongoing training.

Enrichment

The following vignettes illustrate how the lives of just two people have been enriched by their voluntary involvement with the hospice. It is almost overwhelming to consider the vast number of hospice volunteers worldwide in terms of extrapolating the tremendous personal growth and inspiration that has benefited countless numbers of people. This staggering figure can be further multiplied by the numbers of patients, families, and friends who have in turn been able to experience an improved quality of life because of the generosity of hospice volunteers.

> I joined the hospice after working through a traumatic period in my own life. I felt that helping others would help me, which it certainly has done. I have gained knowledge through the very interesting training courses. Working with patients has taught me compassion, humility, and tolerance. As sick as they are, the patients and their families are very grateful for anything one does for them. Their gratitude is touching. I have learned that the few patients who are demanding just need to be listened to and understood. I admire the many dedicated people who work for hospice, both the staff and my fellow volunteers. Sometimes I wonder how the world would ever have managed without the Hospice Movement. (Pam)

I have been a volunteer with South Coast Hospice since the early eighties and have developed experience and a wide knowledge in dealing with terminally ill patients. At first, most of the patients had cancer, particularly of the cervix or oesophagus, lately most of our patients have AIDS. I have gained a greater understanding of community and family dynamics. It is great to enjoy so much respect from the community, they really appreciate my services as a volunteer. Initially, my husband was not sure that my being a volunteer was a good idea but all the positive feedback from the community has made him proud and very supportive of my work. In the beginning I worked in the urban area but was able to be instrumental in getting hospice services to my own outlying rural area. (Nomangesi)

The value of volunteers

In addition to bringing so much 'heart' into a professional organization, the generosity of volunteers allows hospices to extend their service to reach vast numbers of people in need. Without volunteers, many of those in the greatest need might not be able to benefit from the sensitive, holistic palliative care, which hospices in the developing world strive to provide. In sub-Saharan Africa, volunteer care of HIV positive people also has important spin-offs for prevention relative to the rampant HIV/AIDS epidemic. By looking after HIV positive people, caregivers demonstrate to others in the community that there is no risk of becoming infected through everyday contact.[8] They also practise and teach universal precautions as appropriate.

Conclusion

The HIV/AIDS epidemic is presenting hospices in the developing world with enormous challenges and opportunities. Challenges, as these organizations become increasingly reliant on committed, quality volunteer input. Volunteers are a potential human resource which needs to be developed and nurtured. The challenges are accompanied by unprecedented opportunities in terms of the recognition of hospice expertise and credibility. How hospices respond to the escalating needs for palliative care will have a profound effect on individual organizations. It will also affect the future form and course of palliative care as well as its position in the formal health care sector.[9] The fact that government hospitals feel overwhelmed by the demands of the epidemic has undoubtedly contributed greatly to their collaboration with palliative care services which is so necessary for the success of the integrated community-based home care model. Hospices in sub-Saharan Africa are currently in a strong position in terms of impacting on health care policy. The Hospice Association of South Africa is actively lobbying for a quality palliative care component to be included in government home-based care programmes.

Appendix 1
The Hospice Association of South Africa (HASA) audit tool*
Palliative care audit instrument: Client or family interview

Site:_____   Date:_____

Interviewee(s):_____

Choose a client who is bedridden or almost bedridden for this interview, but one who can speak and understand questions.

NR	ITEM	YES	NO
1	Where you given the opportunity to discuss your needs and problems?		
2	Did you feel that these were adequately addressed?		
3	Were you given sufficient information to enable you to understand and plan treatment and care?		
4	Was your pain controlled to your satisfaction?		
5	Were other symptoms controlled to your satisfaction?		
6	Did you receive support from other health professionals when you needed it to meet your needs? NB: This item is also N/A in areas with limited provider options.		
7	Were you referred to other health services when necessary? NB: This item is also N/A in areas where service options are limited.		
8	Have you received sufficient information and training from health care workers to enable you to cope at home? NB: This item is addressed mainly to carers.		
9	Do you know how and where to contact them (community caregivers) if you need assistance?		
10	Do you feel that the health care workers have kept information concerning you and your condition confidential?		

Notes:

NA, not applicable. Use this when an item does not apply to the client, and explain why you do this.

Not Asked, use this when you choose not to ask a specific question (e.g. you cannot ask item 10) if a family member who is not in the confidence of the client is present during the interview.

*Appendices 1–3 have been reproduced by kind permission of the Chief Executive of the Hospice Association of South Africa (HASA).

Appendix 2
Palliative care audit instrument: Palliative care units

Unit:_____ Date:_____ NR of beds:_____

On interview:_____

NR	ITEM	YES	NO
1	TRAINING		
1.1	Is there a written record of In Service Training?		
1.2	Do the records show that at least three levels of health care workers have received in service training over the past two years?		
1.3	Are the following included in the In Service Training Programmes?		
1.3.1	Holistic approach to pain management.		
1.3.2	The WHO Pain Ladder.		
1.3.3	Holistic approach to symptom control.		
1.3.4	Psycho-social care of client and family.		
1.3.5	Spiritual care of client and family.		
1.3.6	Legal and ethical aspects.		
1.3.7	Use of the referral system or network of care.		
1.3.8	Bereavement care.		
1.3.9	Family support.		
1.3.10	Patient advocacy.		
2	RESOURCES		
2	Is there a list of resource organizations and persons including HIV/AIDS resources in the area to whom the client and family may be referred?		
2.2	Is there a named interdisciplinary resource team available for the primary care provider?		
2.3	Is there access to an identified ethics committee.		
2.4	Are there documented methods to access grants and other forms of social assistance? NB: If a social worker is available to take care of these aspects, this is N/A		
2.5	Is there access to medication according to patient needs?		
2.6	Is there a referral form available for use?		
2.7	Are support groups and/or counselling services available for families and significant others?		
2.8	Is counselling available for clients about treatment options, prophylaxis and other issues?		

3	POLICIES AND GUIDELINES		
3.1	Are there written policies on:		
3.1.1	Criteria for access to the care? NB: This refers specifically to which clients are assisted at which services. If these criteria are clear, this gives a YES.		
3.1.2	Infection control?		
3.1.3	Treating health care workers exposed to accidental infections (e.g. needlestick injuries)?		
3.1.4	Handling pain medication (ordering, storage and administration)?		
3.2	Are the following guidelines or protocols available?		
3.2.1	Clinical.		
3.2.2	Psycho-social.		
3.3	Are guidelines reviewed annually?		
3.4	Holistic identification and support of AIDS orphans.		
4	THE CARE TEAM		
4.1	Do members of the care team have access to:		
4.1.1	Structured support programmes in on-duty time? NB: A structured programme refers to regular and scheduled meetings or times.		
4.1.2	Support in coping with illness, dying and bereavement as needed. NB: This item refers to support when the staff needs it.		
4.2	The unit has an adequate skills mix in the staff to cope with client care.		
4.3	Staffing levels makes palliative care possible. NB: this refers specifically to going beyond physical care only.		
4.4	Written job descriptions reflect a palliative care focus.		
4.5	Suitably skilled supervisors to provide support. NB: This refers to a person with palliative care or mental health care training.		
4.6	Does communication in the team enhance care?		
4.7	Are updated treatment guidelines or protocols available to inform staff of recent policies?		
4.8	At least one member of the team is trained in palliative care.		
4.9	Non-professional members form part of the team.		

Record review

NB: Please choose 3 charts for every 10 beds in the unit. Exclude comatose patients.

NR	ITEM	YES	NO
5	Do the records show that:		
5.1	The client and family is the unit of care?		
5.2	The physical needs of the client and family have been identified?		
5.3	The psycho-social needs of the client and family have been identified?		
5.4	The spiritual needs of the client and family have been identified?		
5.5	Pain is managed holistically? NB: There needs to be evidence of interventions other than medication used for pain control for a YES.		
5.6	Pain and other symptoms are managed to the client's satisfaction? NB: There needs to be evidence of patient reaction to nursing intervention showing improvement or satisfaction for a YES.		
5.7	Symptom management is done holistically? NB: There needs to be evidence of interventions other than physical for a YES.		
5.8	The WHO Pain Ladders are used in the management of pain? NB: There needs to be evidence of higher levels of pain control interventions being used in later stages of illness for a YES		
5.9	Each client has a named primary care provider?		
5.10	Therapeutic, psycho-social and spiritual care resources have been mobilized when needed?		
5.11	Is there documentation to show that the client and family, when appropriate, received training in:		
5.11.1	• self-care?		
5.11.2	• Use and side-effects of medication?		
5.12	Are the following charts included in the client record where applicable?		
5.12.1	Pain charts		
5.12.2	Medicine charts		

Appendix 3
Palliative care audit instrument for community services

Site:_____   Date:_____

Choose at least three client records of clients who were not comatose for the main period of care.

NR	ITEM	YES	NO
1	Is there an adequate transport system to enable carers to reach clients?		
2	Is there sufficient equipment for loan/hire for clients?		
3	Are there back-up beds in the community for admissions?		
4	There is a policy or system for follow-up of clients who do not comply with referrals?		
5	In the case of client-held records, is continuity of care recorded?		
6	Do records show that clients have been assisted to continue involvement in life to the limit of his/her capacity?		
7	Is there documentation to show that the client and family receive training in:		
7.1	Self-care?		
7.2	Use and side-effects of medication?		
7.3	Home medicine charts?		
8	Is home charting of medicines accurate?		
9	Supervision.		
9.1	Formal supervision of community caregivers is done.		
9.2	There is evidence of home visits by professional supervisors.		

References

1. Health Systems Trust (HST) (1998). *HST update.* HST, South African National Department of Health, Pretoria.
2. Strachan K, South African Department of Health (SADH) (1998). *SADH report.* South African National Department of Health, Pretoria.
3. Murchison Hospital (1999). Unpublished report. (Available from Murchison Hospital, Port Shepstone, South Coast, Kwazulu-Natal, South Africa).
4. Hunter S (2000). *Reshaping societies: HIV/AIDS and social change,* p. 129. Hudson Run Press, New York.
5. UNAIDS Point of View (1997). *Women and AIDS,* p. 2. UNAIDS, Geneva.
6. UNAIDS (2000). *Report on the global HIV/AIDS epidemic,* p. 37. UNAIDS, Geneva.
7. Campbell L (2001). *Interim Report UGU South HIV/AIDS/STD/TB Pilot Site.* (Unpublished).
8. UNAIDS (2000). *Report on the global HIV/AIDS epidemic,* p. 87. UNAIDS, Geneva.
9. Defilippi K M (2000). Palliative care issues in sub-saharan Africa. *International Journal of Palliative Nursing,* **6(3)**, 108.

Chapter 9

Volunteers working in a tertiary referral teaching hospital

The role of a volunteer working within a tertiary referral hospital palliative care service, although similar in many ways to that of someone working in a free-standing, privately funded or community hospice is quite different in some key areas. Institutional policies, financing, legal restrictions, unions, and differing departmental practices all influence how volunteers are able to function and interact in this setting. This chapter looks at some of these variables and suggests ways to establish and enhance palliative care volunteer programmes in hospital settings. The authors have worked in different teaching hospitals of the same university and their experience at times has been similar and at times, very different, in accord with the culture and community bias of their respective hospitals. These similarities and differences will be highlighted to show the range of options for volunteer co-ordinators to design and implement volunteer palliative care programmes that address the specific needs and cultures of their institutions.

Guiding principles and assumptions

The role of the palliative care volunteer, in any setting, is to provide assistance, companionship, and support to terminally ill patients and their caregiver(s) or families. The aim of their involvement is to enhance the quality of life of the patient or caregiver by offering their time, practical support, commitment, and compassion throughout the illness experience. Our challenge is to offer such support within the complexities and boundaries of a large teaching hospital.

Two guiding principles and assumptions underscore the successful integration of volunteer programmes in hospital palliative care services and form the basis for ongoing communication with members of the professional palliative care team:

1 Volunteer programmes are an essential part of the hospital's palliative care service.

2 Volunteers are essential members of the interdisciplinary palliative care team.

These principles address the central question of whether volunteers are wanted, or needed, and in what capacity. If they are wanted, then by whom? The medical team? The nursing staff? What roles are they needed for? Are there union implications if volunteers are seen to be taking over staff roles, especially in times of budget constraints and downsizing of staff across the health care spectrum? These are difficult and recurring questions for team management and their answers must be clearly established within the palliative care team and must be part of an ongoing dialogue as team members change. Flowing from these principles is a commitment from both the Volunteer Co-ordinator (or Volunteer Service Manager—VSM) and the members of the palliative care team to recognize and include the voice of volunteers in management meetings, decision making, patient rounds, and education programmes for all staff on the service. It is important for the VSM to develop clear standards of practice for volunteer services and to actively participate in quality assessment programmes and working groups within the hospital to ensure that the volunteer voice is heard and recognized as a key input to quality end-of-life care.

Administration: how the programme fits into the wider hospital framework

To whom is the programme accountable? To whom is each service component responsible? How are programme decisions made? What are the lines of reporting? Who controls and sets the budget? How does the programme fit into the wider volunteer framework within the hospital?

In a large teaching hospital, there are several volunteer departments, each with its own co-ordinator and volunteer team. In our hospitals, there are co-ordinators of volunteers in specialized departments, such as oncology, palliative care, emergency department, pastoral services, and there is an overall department of volunteers whose members perform a range of tasks including those in the gift shop, library, out-patient clinics, etc. It is essential that we co-ordinate programmes amongst ourselves to avoid overlap of service but retain continuity of service, for example, when a patient passes from an active treatment floor in oncology to the palliative care unit.

In our respective hospitals, we are responsible to the:

♦ Chief or administrative assistant of the palliative care service for day-to-day administration on the palliative care unit.

♦ Co-ordinator of the volunteer department of the hospital for issues that concern *overall* hospital policies and volunteer activities in the hospital.

We meet regularly with this person on hospital volunteer activities, report monthly on volunteer hours, process all applications through this office, keep them informed of any resignations, address changes, plan 'Volunteer Recognition Days' and activities with them, obtain parking passes, lunch tickets, and smocks and identification badges. This system works very well. It is important that we work with the volunteer department on general volunteer activities, but on issues that are pertinent to the palliative care unit we need to work within the palliative care team, and collaborate with other volunteer departments in the hospital as needed.

The interdisciplinary team/working together

It is the mantra of health care systems that interdisciplinary teams provide the most comprehensive approach to patient care—each team member bringing a perspective and expertise that contributes to an understanding of the whole person. What perspective and expertise does the volunteer bring to this team, and how will that voice be heard?

Whether you are establishing a new volunteer service or maintaining or expanding an existing one, it is essential to obtain an agreement from the palliative care team that volunteers are necessary, and that there is a clear mandate as to their role within the team:

◆ **Establish guidelines for the volunteer programme**—who will do what, when, and how? Will volunteers assist with patient care? Who will train them in this? To whom will volunteers report and how will they access patient information?

◆ **A co-ordinator/manager** (volunteer or paid) **is needed** to recruit, train, supervise, and liaise with volunteers, staff, and hospital administration.

◆ **Examine, review and become familiar with policies within the institution** and its various departments on volunteers. Are there union constraints on what tasks volunteers can perform? Are there legal restrictions, for example, accessing or recording in patient charts? What insurance/liability coverage is available to volunteers who incur an injury on the job?

◆ **New programmes must be negotiated through appropriate channels.** Some are not always transferable; for example, pet therapy may work on one unit and not another for reasons of infection control.

◆ **Volunteers must have ongoing training, support and recognition.** Recurrent debriefing, evaluation and education is essential (by staff, co-ordinator and other volunteers). Regular volunteer meetings provide a forum to discuss cases, share concerns, receive support from peers, and build a strong team.

◆ **Volunteers must be given tools**—information and feedback mechanisms such as tapes, record keeping in notebooks, and direct communication with staff and co-ordinator. They must also be updated on any changes in infection protocols or other floor issues.

◆ **Respect for volunteers from the team** and from volunteers to the team is paramount. Volunteers should be accorded professional courtesies in line with their place on the multidisciplinary team and in turn, they need to follow through with commitment and responsibility to any task or patient to whom they are assigned.

◆ **Develop a scheme to help volunteers cope with change.** Teaching hospitals differ from smaller community hospitals in the frequency of staff changes. Volunteers must cope with frequent shift changes and changes of staff (residents, medical students on a short elective, fellows, research projects, etc.). Ongoing and reciprocal orientation to each other's work is necessary for effective communication.

Volunteers must follow rules, guidelines, and respect boundaries and confidences and these need to be clearly defined at interview and throughout training.

♦ **Clear procedures for airing grievances** and reporting incidents are essential.

♦ **Individual talents and skills must be recognized** and effectively utilized, keeping in mind that volunteers work under volunteer guidelines, not previous or external professional competencies.

♦ **Clarity about financing and funding is essential.** Who is financing the volunteer programme, including salary costs for the co-ordinator/manager, supplies, and materials? In both our hospitals, at present, the palliative care volunteer programme is privately resourced by donors, with office space and some supplies granted by the hospital administration. Fund-raising projects must be cleared with administration. It is imperative to establish clear goals and budget for the service and to work within this constraint.

♦ **Information sharing.** In both our services, patient information comes from the medical and nursing teams, patient charts, and attendance at ward rounds. Only accredited staff (including the volunteer co-ordinator) have access to patient records. (*Volunteers do not read nursing charts on patients and do not record in them.*) How is information about a patient passed to the volunteer? Our systems are different. In one hospital, information is verbally passed to the primary nurse and this is incorporated in a daily tape recording of information and instructions for volunteers which is listened to by all volunteers as they start their shift. In another hospital, volunteers have their own logbook, with separate entries for each patient. Staff have full access to these notes as do subsequent volunteers who can read brief notes about previous volunteer interactions and follow up on any individual requests. The volunteer notes do not form part of the hospital chart. Both systems work equally well, as does a general communication book where volunteers and staff can leave messages and notes to one another. The method of passing information is not prescribed; each co-ordinator and head nurse will determine a method which meets their needs for their unit and team.

♦ It is important that the volunteer co-ordinator meets regularly with unit staff and is involved in issues concerning the unit. A voice not heard is a voice easily overlooked.

Volunteer profile: who are the volunteers?

Volunteers are as mixed and varied as the patients and families they serve. They are the 82-year-old grandmother who has given a lifetime of service to others; the 38-year-old student completing a doctorate in languages; the 58-year-old retired social worker, herself a cancer survivor; the 66-year-old retired pharmacist; the 45-year-old mother returning to university to study psychology; the 56-year-old retired nurse, now a massage therapist; the immigrant mother wanting to help her community; the accountant wanting to work evenings or the medical student wanting experience. Many faces, cultures, religions, and professions—they reflect the make-up of our multicultural and diverse community. Many have been touched by cancer—either personally or a close member of the family. Many have a personal affiliation and loyalty to the hospital where they choose to volunteer—they were born there; their father died there; they see it as their family hospital. Volunteers who are attracted to working in a hospital setting are often more educated and many have had experience in healthcare settings, often in a professional capacity. Many students (particularly of medicine, nursing, and social work) apply to the programme looking for volunteer experience to supplement their résumé. They are often attracted by the prestige of the institution and staff and the educational opportunities to be found at a particular hospital. While their enthusiasm is infectious, they do not always remain with the programme and their class schedules can be a logistical nightmare for the volunteer co-ordinator.

The demographic profile of volunteers has changed in recent years. We do not have as many full-time homemakers who have made volunteering a part of their lives. Nowadays, these women are working and raising a family. We have many more working people who want to volunteer in the evenings and weekends (the co-ordinator usually works day shifts). Again, their schedules change frequently and they are often absent because of work or travel. More men are volunteering, but we need more. Many retirees now spend a significant part of the winter in warmer climates, thus also leaving gaps in scheduling and consistency of service. It is a constant challenge to recruit and retain a volunteer team which truly reflects the diversity of our patients and which will give reliable and consistent service without constantly amending the schedule.

We also attract many retired professionals. Among our volunteers we have retired physicians, social workers, physiotherapists, psychologists, nurses, a speech therapist, massage therapists and business executives. From the outset it is necessary to fully explain that they must set their professional 'cap' aside. They are not there to mediate, diagnose, treat, or give advice, but to offer compassion and support. They are required to follow our rules and guidelines. Generally, they say they are relieved to not carry the responsibility of a professional, but happy just to accompany the patient and family—a luxury they did not have in a professional capacity.

In our hospitals, it would not be possible for an active health care professional to work, in their professional capacity, as a volunteer, with the exception of some complementary therapists, such as a massage therapist or aromatherapist. These therapists often donate a few hours per week, and in both our hospitals receive referrals receive referrals from the medical and nursing teams, via the head nurse or the VSM. They are art of the volunteer service and subject to the same screening, as well as their professional qualifications would be accepted by the Chief of the Division. While health professionals do not work as volunteers, it must be said that everyone on the team—doctors, nurses, psychologists, etc., regularly work hours over and above their paid duties, come to the hospital after-hours or on days off to sit with a patient, attend a celebration which is meaningful to a family or to make condolence visits. While they are not volunteers in any literal sense, they share much in spirit. It is what makes a good team work—knowing that team members will do what is necessary in the interests of patients and their colleagues.

Recruitment and selection of volunteers

Selection must be thorough and careful as in all palliative care settings. Special considerations in a teaching hospital setting are:

♦ Recruitment should target a good representative mix of ages, cultures, experience, and languages if possible to meet the needs of patients in a multicultural hospital.

♦ Volunteers in a hospital setting must be team players and respect boundaries, guidelines of the programme, institution, and departments.

♦ Volunteers need to be screened and accepted both by the palliative care VSM and the co-ordinator of volunteers for the hospital. The initial interview provides the opportunity for the co-ordinator to explore and assess the applicant's motives, expectations, suitability, and stability. There are many motivations for volunteering in a palliative unit, including the wish to 'give back' if their loved one had the experience of receiving good palliative care or wanting to give to others what had not been available to them when they needed it. Some feel it is part of their own personal growth journey. Our aim, as volunteer co-ordinators, is to ensure that an applicant's personal agenda, including their religious beliefs or a need to ease past losses, does not interfere with, or compromise, a patient's well-being and personal values. In our hospitals, a police check is also required.

♦ Volunteers must wear appropriate identification at all times—smock or coat and name badge.

A day in the life of a volunteer in Montreal: what do they do?

Assuming the volunteer has passed the initial interview and completed the compulsory training programme, what is expected of them on any given day?

♦ First and foremost, they listen. They are there for the patient and family to support them in any way possible. A conversation, accompaniment in silence, a gentle hand or foot massage, tidying the room, offering a cup of tea—all are small ways to ease the burden of the patient or family member and provide a moment of 'normality' in an otherwise noisy and busy hospital environment.

♦ Assist the nurse with patient care. Volunteers are assigned in the morning to work with the nurses helping to change beds, give bed baths, showers, and whirlpool baths, help with feeding (from delivery of trays to total feeding), personal care, toileting, transferring, massage, etc. Volunteers are kept informed about 'do's and don'ts' by means of a comprehensive daily report from the nurse.

♦ Transfers are *never* done alone, and all care is done under the supervision of the nurse. Training is provided in areas of transfers, feeding, infection control, and mobilization. Volunteers *never* give medication or do any medical interventions (injections, dressing changes, catheter insertions, etc.). However, they are often present to assist in some way (holding hands, supporting the patient, fetching supplies, handing the nurse equipment, etc.).

◆ Take patients for a walk or in a wheelchair, or help with recreation and hobbies, where appropriate.

◆ Provide respite to a tired caregiver. Volunteers may sit with a patient while a caregiver goes for lunch or runs personal errands.

◆ Provide a link to the team. Volunteers often hear and see things that may be relevant to the patient's care plan, particularly how much pain is being experienced or expressed to staff—'they're so busy!' A volunteer may encourage the patient to report symptoms or pain to the doctor, or with their permission, pass on relevant information to staff. Volunteers have an important advocacy role both for patients and families.

Volunteers bring care, compassion, and companionship to those to whom they are assigned. They bring themselves—their personalities, quirks, stories, experience, wit, and wisdom and mostly they bring the gift of time. In a busy tertiary referral teaching hospital where staff rush from patient to patient and complaints about 'not having enough time' to spend with patients are common, volunteers take the time to make a difference in someone's day. It is not uncommon for volunteers to do special things for a patient, bring in a video of a hockey game to watch with a patient, help someone make a scrapbook, teach someone to knit or to bring special treats and homemade goodies. Sometimes a patient needs to be careful what he/she wishes for—a loose remark of 'I just want some chicken soup' soon has the unit awash in chicken soup as each volunteer brings enough to start a small restaurant. Staff can eat very well sometimes from the generosity of volunteers!

Volunteers help with the many personal events and celebrations on the palliative care unit. We have assisted and witnessed many birthdays, holiday celebrations, baptisms, bar mitzvahs, and weddings—each helping a patient or family member achieve a meaningful goal in their life. Volunteers provide music, food, and any special assistance to make the event personal and memorable. Most events are small in size, but recently we had a full wedding reception, highlighting the need for co-operation between multiple departments of the hospital to make it happen. One of our patients wanted to see the last of his children married and it was obvious that he would not live to the pre-planned date. The family decided to bring the wedding forward and have the ceremony and a small reception on the unit. Some sixty guests were planned and this could not be accommodated on the unit. So, quick planning between the volunteers, the hospital chaplain, housekeeping, recreation, and the nursing staff on the geriatrics unit resulted in a wedding being held on this unit, where there was more space, and a full wedding, complete with bridesmaids, photographer, caterers, and a three-piece band was possible. We were able to help a very proud father witness and give blessings to the marriage of his daughter, enjoy a dance in his bed with his wife and daughter and to capture the moment for future generations. It was a day of grace and love, and it brought together staff and volunteers from different services who were also blessed by the moment.

Volunteers do not plan weddings on an everyday basis!—but they are part of many small meaningful moments for patients and their families. It is what they do best and for what they are most appreciated, and it is always a surprise what might happen on any given day.

Where do the volunteers work?

Volunteers work all over the hospital, in every department and clinic. The volunteers in the wider hospital fall under the supervision of the Co-ordinator of Volunteers for the hospital who has a separate staff. There are many volunteer activities from a 'cuddles programme' in the neonatal department to volunteers in the transplant and dialysis departments. All require separate applications and training programmes and generally there is no integration of volunteers.

Palliative care volunteers must apply, be accepted and be trained to be part of the palliative care team. They work in the following areas.

Palliative care unit

Volunteers work primarily on the unit itself—a 16–17 bed-dedicated unit. Shifts are normally four hours each, although some volunteers choose to work longer hours. Morning, afternoon and evening shifts are offered, seven days a week.

Oncology floors

Palliative care volunteers are not loaned to other departments when there is a shortfall or high need, but palliative care volunteers do visit patients on other floors, at the referral of the consulting team. These patients are often on a waiting list for admission to the palliative unit, and it significantly reduces the stress of patients and families to know a familiar face and have a relationship with a volunteer if the patient is ultimately admitted to the unit. Many families tell us it made all the difference and allayed a great deal of fear about the unit itself. Sometimes, the referral is for a patient who will remain on another floor, at the recommendation of their physician, even if a bed on the unit becomes available. In this case, the volunteer would 'visit' and provide support, perhaps assist with feeding, but would not be part of the team on that floor, *per se*. The volunteer is part of the palliative care team, in this case providing outreach to a patient on another floor.

Bereavement outreach

Some volunteers also work in bereavement outreach and support programmes. Volunteers who have themselves experienced a loss and have completed special training, may be matched with a newly bereaved person and call them at regular intervals over a period of twelve months, until the first anniversary of the death.

Other volunteers, also specially trained, co-lead bereavement support groups which are offered in eight-week sessions several times a year. The bereavement volunteers receive referrals, support, and direction from a bereavement co-ordinator, who may be the same person as the Palliative Care Co-ordinator (VSM), or not. Both models exist in our hospitals. The important factor is that bereavement is seen as an essential part of the palliative care programme and volunteers are a key element of the service.

Ecumenical memorial services

In conjunction with pastoral services, a memorial service is offered on the palliative care unit, at intervals appropriate for the institution, for families who have lost a loved one. Volunteers and staff are invited to this service and volunteers play an active role in hosting a tea at the end of the service. Members of the bereavement team are present to assist families, especially those who are alone or seem isolated in their grief.

Training and ongoing education

Training is the cornerstone of the volunteer programme and provides it with credibility and professionalism. It is compulsory for all volunteers to complete a comprehensive training programme *before* they start work on the service. (See the Appendix 1.) It changes a little from year to year to reflect new topics and concerns. For example, 'Ethics' and 'Complementary Therapies' are relatively recent additions. In addition, there is an expectation that volunteers will avail themselves of regular in-house education opportunities to enhance their skills. Further areas of training include:

♦ Practical training in admission criteria for palliative care, diseases involved, treatment options, DNR (Do Not Resuscitate) orders, hydration, feeding, palliative surgery, radiotherapy and chemotherapy, infection control procedures, transfers, feeding, personal hygiene care, and mobilization techniques.

♦ Volunteers must be thoroughly oriented to working on the unit and in other departments in the hospital. This can be done by an experienced volunteer.

♦ A clearly defined probation period, mentoring with an experienced volunteer, and scheduled time with the VSM for debriefing and feedback are important training practices.

♦ In our services, the formal training programme is usually provided by professionals on the palliative care service. During the year, staff may also be invited to lecture to the volunteers on a given topic, and volunteers are always invited to university palliative care rounds or to hear visiting lecturers. Volunteers are very much included in educational activities and conferences which provide networking opportunities with other volunteers from different settings.

♦ Volunteer team meetings once a month are another rich source of training and support.

Training for staff

Training must also be provided for staff to sensitize them to working with volunteers. This is an extremely important area and one which is often overlooked. In a teaching hospital, this needs to be done on a frequent basis to accommodate changing rotations of residents and medical students.

Common problems and special issues

Having briefly highlighted some of the factors necessary to establish and maintain a professionally accepted and professional volunteer programme in a large teaching hospital, we now look at some of the most common problems we have encountered in co-ordinating our teams:

◆ *Selecting and retaining appropriate volunteers*—often the most keen, enthusiastic applicants are those who do not last—the job does not meet the expectations they had of it, or their personal schedule is too demanding to allow consistency of volunteering. During the interview and the training one can weed out some inappropriate volunteers, and the probation period provides a good opportunity for close supervision.

◆ *Finding appropriate tasks for volunteers who have special skills and experience,* including using them as mentors or buddies to other volunteers. Developing a skills' bank is one way to keep track of the special talents of individual volunteers.

◆ *Juggling schedules and being flexible enough to accommodate volunteers' schedules*—some volunteers are away for the whole summer, or the whole winter, students' schedules change frequently, volunteers take vacations or are sick.

◆ *Finding creative ways to train volunteers* and to keep the in-house education updated and appropriate to the knowledge and skill level of the volunteers, especially for veteran volunteers with many years of experience.

◆ *Providing ongoing feedback and support to volunteers to enhance their skills.* This can be a full-time job in itself, but one which pays huge dividends in retaining volunteers and preventing major disciplinary problems.

◆ *Recognizing and dealing with grief and potential 'burn-out'* of team members—providing support, a leave of absence, if appropriate, and follow-up.

◆ *Increasing the demand for volunteer services only to find there are not sufficient volunteers* or conversely, having too many volunteers and not enough work. This is a rare occurrence but speaks to the need for ongoing communication with the palliative care team to ensure that staff, particularly new staff, are aware of the volunteer's role and relevant availability and can therefore make appropriate requests for volunteers to assist with a patient or family member.

◆ *Expanding and developing the volunteer programme when professional staff are being 'downsized' by the institution as a result of budget constraints.* This is a new challenge for VSMs and it will only increase as health systems undergo reform and change. The possibility of 'turf wars' is an area of great sensitivity and requires honest communication, trust, and clear definition of roles and responsibilities within the whole palliative care team. It may be necessary to meet with union representation if a threat to their jobs is perceived.

• In many ways, it is an anomaly to have a palliative care unit in an acute care hospital, where the ethos is cure, rapid processing of patients, and releasing beds as soon as possible. Volunteers working on the palliative unit are somewhat protected from this pressure, but it is certainly felt on oncology floors where patients are treated, discharged, and readmitted as needed. It is more difficult to build relationships with the patients and families and the volunteer may pass by the room many times before connecting with a patient who is having tests or treatment. Even on the palliative care unit, there may be multiple admissons as a patient's pain and symptoms are managed (sometimes with radiation, chemotherapy or surgery for palliative relief of the symptoms); the patient may go home for a while and be readmitted if the symptoms again cause a level of distress that cannot be managed with home care.

In our hospitals today, there is often a shortage of nurses and beds, and there are long waiting lists, including for palliative care. Volunteers can and do find this stressful at times, but it is the role of the VSM to debrief with volunteers they assess as being noticeably stressed or at risk of burn-out, and 'Taking Care of Oneself' is a training module repeated as often as required.

Dismissing a volunteer

Dealing with volunteers who overstep guidelines and boundaries can be challenging. Is it ever necessary to dismiss a volunteer? Have we ever had to do so? If a volunteer were to overstep a boundary (e.g. giving aromatherapy to a patient without approval), we would sit with that volunteer to explain the implications of doing this and to re-emphasize the importance of following the rules and checking with the staff before doing so. There may be allergies, respiratory problems, etc., of which the volunteer is unaware. Generally, this would be sufficient, and can be set in a context of ongoing training and support for the volunteer. However, if it happened again it would be much more serious and the volunteer would probably be asked to leave.

It is seldom necessary to dismiss volunteers but volunteers may be counselled to leave if they are becoming over-involved with patients and not having a clear sense of personal boundaries. This may indicate unresolved issues or loss in their own past and the emotional nature of palliative care work may not suit them. A different volunteer experience, in a less stressful part of the hospital or community may be more suited to their needs. Sometimes, we recommend a volunteer take a leave of absence from the programme to prevent burn-out and take some time for themselves.

We would ask a volunteer to leave if they have been consistently unreliable in reporting for work. Usually, this indicates a lack of enthusiasm or availability for the job and as we generally have a waiting list for volunteer positions, we will give the spot to another. In many years it has not happened very often. We start with the assumption that the volunteer is well-intentioned and we find that good screening, training, mentoring by an experienced volunteer and ongoing communication and support for the volunteer during the probation period works well and prevents most problems becoming major ones.

Challenges and opportunities for the VSM

Health care is changing; downsizing is a reality, and the volunteer role is more important than ever. VSMs are faced with great challenges and opportunities to introduce innovative programmes to supplement those of the medical and nursing teams. But it can be a lonely job, often poorly financed, if at all, and with many more tasks to fill the day than hours allowed. We offer a few suggestions that have helped us in our work and have offered us inspiration, joy, and challenge.

Network with others

This is possibly the single most effective way to broaden your perspective and experience. Link with other volunteer co-ordinators in your community—hospitals, hospices, and community health programmes. Meet on a regular basis (e.g. every other month), and share programme ideas, upcoming workshops and seminars, challenges and concerns, and even more importantly, your successes. The support of your peers is enriching and invaluable and in a very practical sense, can save you time and money by sharing resources, advertising each other's workshops, and developing some common training materials. The network does not need to be exclusively palliative care. In Montreal, we have developed a rich network of volunteer co-ordinators/VSMs from oncology day programmes as well as those in palliative care. Where the opportunity does not exist for personal contact with other co-ordinators, this can be done on-line, for example. The important thing is to link with others and share ideas and experience.

Share the training

As above, there is much to be gained by sharing resources, expenses, and ideas with other co-ordinators. In recent years, we have joined with the co-ordinator of another hospital in Montreal and the three of us have devised a common training programme, based on the standards of the Canadian Palliative Care Association. Similar standards are available in many countries. We have presented this material in three different formats to meet the needs of our hospitals and the volunteer applicants:

+ a two day weekend workshop;
+ a four evening workshop (two evenings per week);
+ a two day mid-week workshop.

Each hospital provided trainers and volunteers, and material costs were shared. Each of these formats was highly interactive and experiential in design. Role-plays, discussions, and hands-on practice of hygiene care, for example, were key features. These inter-hospital programmes supplemented existing lecture-based training in each hospital. Feedback from participants showed that the inter-hospital format was highly successful in encouraging networking, and exploring differences between hospitals, particularly cultural and religious differences between some individual programmes and the differences in roles performed by the volunteers in different settings. Some were more hands-on, assisting with bed care and personal hygiene, with other hospitals adopting a more 'friendly visitor' role for their volunteers.

Sharing training also meant that more volunteers could be trained on a regular basis, rather than each hospital waiting until they had 'enough' to justify the expense of running their own training programme. A further benefit was that it met volunteers' personal needs more quickly—they were able to start work sooner, and could get a training programme to suit their hours. Full-time workers appreciated the evening or weekend schedules, and others, particularly retired people, appreciated the day-time hours.

Be informed

Read current journals and articles. There is a growing wealth of literature in volunteer management in general, both in print and on the Internet. Explore relevant websites for free ideas on training, management, program design, and volunteer recognition ideas, to name but a few. Contribute to on-line discussions about your work and learn from others in similar settings.

Use the resources of the team

Although the interdisciplinary team model is so prized, its full resources are often not used, and problem-solving in isolation is common. Fellow team members may have a perspective, experience, and insight that are valuable and relevant to the issue you are dealing with, whether it be training, discipline, administration, scheduling or emotional support for yourself or one of your volunteer team. Use your team members—it builds trust, camaraderie, and interdependence—as well as possibly solving your problem. Equally, valuable resources exist within your volunteer team. Use them. It is an excellent way to identify potential leaders, mentors and trainers.

Participate in hospital committees and rounds

Teaching hospitals abound in committees and working groups. The volunteer voice is best heard when it is part of multidisciplinary committees—for example, committees and working groups on Palliative Care Standards, Bereavement, Quality of Life, Pastoral Care, and Humanization of Care, and is most easily overlooked when it is not represented. The VSM should be involved, participating actively in ward rounds and ad hoc meetings of ward personnel.

Take advantage of teaching opportunities

One thing teaching hospitals obviously do is teach, and there are many opportunities for VSMs to contribute. They can offer to present the volunteer perspective and role at orientations for new nurses and residents. This is a valuable and ongoing opportunity for dialogue with other disciplines, as staff regularly change rotations in a teaching facility. Present a case at rounds or take advantage of Theme weeks such as Volunteer Week, Palliative Care Week, Humanization of Care Week, etc., to present the volunteer perspective. The organizing committees of such events are always looking for lectures, seminars, and workshops of interest, and it is both a challenge and an opportunity for volunteers to have their voice heard.

In the same vein, participate in local, national, and international conferences where possible, and advocate for a volunteer forum as part of the conference agenda. Networking, teaching, and learning with others is a rich way to broaden one's knowledge and contribute to a developing field of practice wisdom. Encourage volunteers to attend, if the budget allows, and have them present their learning to the next team meeting or write a summary for the team newsletter.

Plan for the future

An annual review of goals and objectives, both for the programme as well as for individual volunteers allows the VSM to keep focus on what is needed to develop his/her programme as well as to devise a strategy to raise funds or solicit donors, as necessary. Have a 'Vision Day'—put on some 3-dimensional glasses and discover if you are seeing clearly! Are you meeting the needs of the unit, the volunteers (how do you know—have you asked them lately?) Evaluations and surveys (formal or informal) are extremely important and informative. Are you meeting your own needs? What needs to change, if anything?

Follow the **3D** approach:

♦ **Delete** when necessary.

♦ **Delegate** whenever possible.

♦ **Dream** about the day when volunteer departments are adequately funded and resourced and you can take it easy!

Conclusion

Despite its sometimes difficult moments, the authors of this chapter have rarely been disenchanted with their work. It has been a joy and a privilege to work in this field and it will become only richer and more exciting as VSMs share their skills and experience and help develop global standards for our work. It is a challenge and a great opportunity for us all.

Appendix 1 A typical training programme (names of speakers deleted)

Volunteer Training Programme—2001

This training program is open to all new and current Palliative Care Service and McGill affiliated hospital staff and Volunteers and interested members of the public.

SESSION I: THURSDAY, SEPTEMBER 20, 2001
6:30–7:30   *The Role of the Volunteer*
7:45–9:00   *The Philosophy of Palliative Care*

SESSION II: THURSDAY, SEPTEMBER 27, 2001
6:30–7:30   *Nursing in Palliative Care*
7:45–9:00   *Pain Management*

SESSION III   THURSDAY, OCTOBER 4, 2001
6:30–7:30   *Families Facing Death*
7:45–9:00   *Music Therapy in Palliative Care*

SESSION IV   THURSDAY, OCTOBER 11, 2001
6:30–7:30   *Quality of Life for Palliative Care Patients and Their Families*
7:45–9:00   *Pastoral Care for Palliative Patients and Their Families*

SESSION V: THURSDAY, OCTOBER 18, 2001
6:30–7:30   *Bereavement Follow-Up in Palliative care*
7:45–9:00   *The Volunteer Experience*

SESSION VI: THURSDAY, OCTOBER 25, 2001
6:30–7:30   *Occupational Therapy in Palliative Care*
7:45–9:00   *Complimentary and Alternative Therapies in Palliative Care*

SESSION VII: THURSDAY, NOVEMBER 1, 2001
6:30–7:30   *Ethics in Palliative Care*
7:45–9:00   *Psychology in Palliative Care*

Chapter 10

Volunteers in a children's hospice

Children's hospices can benefit significantly from the involvement of volunteers. They have much to offer in terms of skills, experience, and time. Enhancing the expertise of the paid staff team, they allow hospices to offer so much more to children and families.

Volunteers, however, do not just happen and the development of a service should not be left to chance. Volunteers need the same supervision and guidance as paid staff but this must be delivered in a very different way. The management task is considerable and is not ideally tacked on to an already busy role. The secret of effective management is that the service is organized with great precision, but is portrayed to the volunteers in a relaxed and friendly way.

An introduction to children's hospices

Children's hospices were set up to offer palliative respite care and terminal care to children with a life-limiting or life-threatening condition.[1] Care extends to the whole family and may be offered in the hospice and in the child's home, extending beyond the death of the child into bereavement support for the family. Children of all ages may be cared for from tiny babies to young people in their early twenties.

Within a children's hospice, as in adult hospices, the emphasis is on living and helping to make the most of the time children have left. Hospices are well equipped with play facilities for children and there are opportunities to play and take part in activities or just to have some quiet time and relaxation. Multisensory rooms, jacuzzis, and 'soft' playrooms are just some of the specialist facilities found in a children's hospice.

When children are first diagnosed with a life-limiting condition or when curative treatment becomes unsuccessful, many families experience fear, loneliness, and a huge sense of loss. As the child's condition progresses, families find themselves under enormous strain. Simple things such as a good night's sleep, shopping or even taking children to the park become difficult, if not impossible. Family life necessarily revolves round the needs of the affected child and siblings often feel left out. Indeed, some families have more than one affected child. Most children's hospices offer accommodation for parents and siblings in order that the whole family can be together and supported during their stay. This is one way in which children's hospices differ from their adult counterparts.

The average number of admissions in one year will vary depending on the size of the hospice and the population served but is approximately 391. The length of stay likewise is dependent on the reason for admission and may vary from hospice to hospice but on average is between three and five nights.

Types of conditions the children suffer from

Children's hospices care for children and young people with a wide range of conditions. In general, less than 11% of them have cancer. The conditions fall into several categories:

- Life-threatening conditions for which curative treatment may be feasible but can fail (e.g cancer, irreversible organ failure).
- Conditions where premature death is possible or inevitable (e.g. Duchenne muscular dystrophy, cystic fibrosis).
- Progressive conditions without the option of curative treatment (e.g Batten's disease, mucopolysaccharidosis, Creutzfeldt – Jakob—CJD disease).
- Severe neurological disability which may cause weakness and susceptibility to health complications (e.g. severe cerebral palsy, severe disabilities following brain or spinal cord injuries).

The environment of a children's hospice

Although the philosophy of children's hospices is very similar to that of an adult unit the environment is very different. Children are seldom to be found in bed. Even when very ill, they may spend much of the day in the main social areas surrounded by other children and the hustle and bustle of the hospice. Because it is important for the atmosphere to be that of 'home-from-home' there is little structure to the day, with care patterns following those of the child whilst at home. Staff generally do not wear uniforms and it can be hard to distinguish staff from parents or volunteers. Many parents are surprised on their first visit to be met with siblings running about and young people in electric wheelchairs moving at high speed. The atmosphere is filled with children's noise and laughter.

There are however profoundly sad times when a death occurs. In contrast to an adult hospice, children, although suffering from a continually deteriorating condition, may die quite suddenly and unexpectedly of an acute problem such as an infection. Not all deaths take place in the hospice, but even if the child dies in hospital or at home, often it is possible for both the child and the family to come to the hospice to stay whilst funeral arrangements are made.

The number of beds varies from hospice to hospice. Some have as few as four whilst others as many as ten. The average number of beds of a children's hospice in the United Kingdom is approximately eight.

Reasons for admission

There may be a variety of reasons for the admission of a child and these may include:

- worsening of the child's condition;
- helping carers adjust to a new treatment regimen;
- illness of the main carer;
- child entering the terminal stage of the illness;
- respite admission to give family a break.

Why involve volunteers?

So why should volunteers be involved in a children's hospice? Although the tradition of volunteering in children's hospices is not as strong as in the adult sector, volunteers have at least as much to offer in the many aspects of a children's service.

First, they form strong links between the communities where they live and the hospice itself, helping to raise awareness and increase understanding of the work of children's hospices. There are still many misconceptions about the work of these hospices and volunteers have a valuable role to play in dispelling myths. Volunteers bring a wide diversity of skills and life experience which enhances that of the paid staff, allowing the hospice to offer so much more to the children and families for whom it cares. They are not so deeply involved with the problems of the families and bring with them a fresh approach. Volunteers are one of the hospices' greatest resources. They are also exemplary ambassadors for their work.

Volunteer roles

There are many areas that can benefit from the involvement of volunteers and the following list is only an indication of some of these areas:

- helping staff to prepare and serve meals;
- helping in reception to answer telephones and welcome visitors to the hospice;
- assisting with typing, filing, and photocopying;
- housekeeping;
- gardening;
- driving—bringing families in to stay in the hospice or taking them out during their visit;
- hairdressing;
- assisting with general maintenance;
- complementary therapies;
- hydrotherapy pool aides;
- befriending children and parents;

+ bereavement befriending;
+ helping with siblings;
+ fund-raising;
+ public speaking—specially trained volunteers giving talks to groups about the work of the hospice.

Good practice recommends that volunteers should not be involved in any aspects of clinical work nor should they be asked to undertake any unpleasant jobs which staff would not carry out themselves.

Planning for volunteer involvement

In deciding to involve volunteers in a children's hospice, the first step should be to develop a policy outlining the hospice's philosophy of volunteering and approach to their involvement. It is important to be clear about what volunteers will be expected to do or not to do and which member of staff will be appointed to be responsible for recruitment and selection, induction, training, support, rostering, review, and management, and smooth running of the volunteer programme. For a voluntary service to be effective, it cannot be left to chance. Volunteers deserve as much guidance support and service planning as paid members of staff.

To be truly representative, volunteers selected should reflect the hospice and local communities in terms of age range, backgrounds, and ethnic origin. In some hospices, a typical age range for volunteers is between 16 and 75 plus.

Before recruitment takes place it is important to assess the types of roles that volunteers will be asked to undertake. Are they motivating, interesting, and varied? Role descriptions should be drawn up for each area of work, outlining the tasks to be undertaken, expectations, support, and supervision offered. This helps to clarify volunteer roles for staff and to give volunteers a clear idea of what they may be expected to do.

It is also helpful to identify the likely number of volunteers required, the skills needed to undertake these roles, and days and times. This helps in deciding the best method of recruitment to employ.

Care must be taken, however, in the wording of all documentation relating to volunteers. Legal problems can ensue if volunteers can be deemed to have a contract and thus to be unpaid employees (see Chapter 13 on legal issues).

The recruitment process begins with the search for prospective volunteers. This continues through matching prospective volunteers' expectations with the needs of the hospice to allow volunteers to make an informed application. There are many different methods of recruiting volunteers (see Chapter 4 on the selection of volunteers), and the search for prospective volunteers is no different in a children's hospice environment.

It must be borne in mind throughout all stages of recruitment and selection, however, that working in a children's hospice environment is particularly challenging. Death of children in society today is, thankfully, uncommon but working in an environment where children die can be at times an extremely emotional experience. It is not the best place for vulnerable people nor those who have recently experienced the death of a loved one, especially the loss of a child. Working with children also requires flexibility and the ability to be prepared to change plans to meet the needs and wishes of children.

Matching expectations and applications

Many prospective volunteers, however, have misconceptions about the nature and work of a children's hospice. It is also the case that if a hospice has a very high profile in the community, there may be an overwhelming number of applications from people wishing to become volunteers. In this instance, a waiting list of prospective volunteers is necessary and this can be a valuable resource to which to return when vacancies do occur.

Those making enquiries may also have unrealistic ideas about the voluntary work they may be able to undertake. A significant number of people come forward wishing to read stories or play with the children. Whilst there may be opportunities for volunteers to be involved in these activities it may be that the hospice really needs help in other areas. It is important, therefore, to take time with would-be volunteers in an information-giving session to talk about the hospice, the care offered there, how volunteers are involved, where volunteers are currently needed, and the recruitment process. This helps in matching volunteers' expectations with the needs of the hospice and allows potential volunteers to self-select at this stage. This information can be given either after the initial enquiry or after receipt of a completed application form.

Time taken at the point of recruiting volunteers is time well spent and experience has shown that this results in good retention rates.

Applications

Once completed, application forms are received, the process of matching skills with vacant volunteer roles can begin before inviting volunteers for interview to explore further their suitability. Volunteers should always be recruited for specific tasks. It causes ambiguity both for volunteers and for staff if volunteers are first recruited and then found 'something to do'. When this situation arises, the volunteer often does not know what they have come to the hospice to do and staff do not know what to ask them to do. The outcome of this is a frustrated volunteer who leaves and a member of staff who then believes that volunteers are at best ineffective and unreliable. Key qualities of a volunteer in a children's hospice are the abilities to be completely flexible and to respond to the changing needs of the children and families. Sometimes, those who have been used to a very structured working environment find adapting to the relaxed atmosphere difficult.

The selection process

It is vital in any hospice that appropriate volunteers are selected for each role in terms of temperament, skills, motivation or ability to undertake the required role.

In a children's hospice it is especially important to explore carefully with prospective volunteers their motivation for volunteering to work with children, attitude to children and experience of young people whether in a paid, voluntary or family capacity.

The purpose of selection is to build up a picture of the prospective volunteer, and to make the right match of personality, skills, and experience (or ability to learn the skills) and to make a good match between the person and the role. It is also intended to identify any person who is clearly unsuitable.

The interview

This is a very important part of the selection process. Interviews should involve the Voluntary Services Manager (VSM) and another member of staff. This should be someone who will supervising or working with the volunteer, as it is important to ensure that they have the opportunity to assess whether the prospective volunteer has the necessary skills and temperament for their area of work. It is important to keep interviews informal and friendly and it is helpful to have a format, for example, a volunteer interview form (see Appendix 1). At the interview the following areas should be explored:

- motivation/s for volunteering with a children's hospice;
- expectations of voluntary work;
- hobbies and interests;
- their interest in, attitudes to, and experience of children;
- experience of loss and bereavement;
- exploration of how they feel they might cope when faced with the loss of a child they have come to know well;
- health;
- times available for voluntary work;
- preference for type of volunteer role (e.g. office or befriending).

The interview also gives an opportunity for prospective volunteers to ask questions and gain a better insight into the children's hospice environment. It is good practice for volunteers wishing to work directly with children, to undergo a second interview which focuses on their motivations for working with children and their attitudes and approach to children (see Appendix 2).

Criminal Records Office checks

The following information is written from a UK perspective and further information can be obtained from the Volunteer Centre UK.[3] Whether in the UK or elsewhere, current legal advice should be sought as legislation may change from time to time.

It is essential to carry out a criminal record check on all volunteers applying to work in a children's hospice as they will have substantial access to children. Because of the nature of this work volunteers would be required by the Rehabilitation of Offenders Act 1974 to declare all criminal convictions including those which are 'spent'. The current system has been reviewed in recent years and police checks are to be called 'Disclosures'. Three levels of Disclosure will be available to organizations:

1 Enhanced Disclosure.

2 Standard Disclosure.

3 Basic Disclosure.

Enhanced and Standard Disclosures have been available in the UK from winter 2001 but only to organizations who fit the criteria. This timescale may change and it is advised that further information should be sought.

1 Enhanced Disclosure

This will:

+ contain details of all current or spent convictions, cautions, reprimands or warnings;
+ identify whether the individual is deemed by the Department of Education and Skills and the Department of Health (or their equivalents) to be unsuitable to work with children;
+ include any other relevant information held by the police will also be included.

2 Standard Disclosure

This will:

+ give the same information as for Enhanced Disclosure but without the addition of extra information held by police.

3 Basic Disclosure

This disclosure contains:

+ details of 'unspent' convictions under the Rehabilitation of Offenders Act.

Selection criteria

It is important to be clear about what qualities to look for in prospective volunteers and what would cause someone to be unsuccessful in their application. Selection criteria might include:

+ genuine interest in the hospice's work;
+ clear reasons/motivation for volunteering (e.g. time to give, to develop confidence, to gain experience for work, to give something back, to make friends, being a few of the most common, interest in children);
+ people who like people, especially children, and can work as part of a team;
+ approachable, flexible people;
+ an empathy for the work of the hospice;
+ tact and sensitivity;

- clear commitment and reliability;
- appropriate skills for the task/s or ability and willingness to learn these;
- clear criminal record check;
- people who have not experienced a recent bereavement, most especially of a child, and who would have the ability to work around loss and bereavement.

Experience has shown that most applicants prove to be suitable and are likely to be accepted as volunteers. Generally, this is attributable to the fact that they have given a great deal of thought before making an application and in the early stages of recruitment have had the opportunity to develop a clearer understanding of the hospice and the role of volunteers. From time to time, however, it will be necessary to turn down a prospective volunteer. Some of the reasons for doing so would include:

- interviewers cannot be sure of the reason/s for wanting to work with children;
- someone who had been convicted of an offence against a child;
- an inappropriate attitude to disability or to children;
- refusal to undergo the Criminal Records Office check;
- an immature young person;
- a recent bereavement, or unresolved loss, especially loss of a child.

Bereavement

Often, people who have been recently bereaved see working in a hospice as a way of helping themselves to resolve their loss. However, working in a situation of frequent loss and bereavement serves only to reawaken experiences and cause further distress.[3] People struggling themselves with a bereavement are also less able to support families and children facing loss.

Introductory training and support

Volunteer induction, like staff induction, is a process rather than an event and ideally takes place over the first three months of a volunteer's involvement with the hospice.

The stages of induction may include:

- first day meeting with the Voluntary Services Manager (VSM) and member of staff with whom the volunteer will be working;
- familiarization with the hospice layout;
- buddying or mentoring with an experienced volunteer;
- learning about the role;
- induction training programme including: information about the hospice's organizational structure, hospice philosophy, what the care means to a family, brief overview of children's conditions, child protection, fund-raising, health and safety awareness, volunteering guidelines, and expectations;
- end of induction review.

The end of induction review is important to hear feedback from the volunteer on their experiences and to give feedback on their performance. If problems have been identified either by the volunteer or the hospice it is important that they are resolved at this point rather than let more time go by. It may be that additional training or a change of role is all that is required to remedy the situation. On rare occasions, however, it may be clear that the hospice is not the right place for the volunteer and it may be necessary to end the relationship.

Support and supervision

Support for everyone who works in a children's hospice environment is vitally important in order to prevent 'burn-out'. The work can be emotionally draining and volunteers are just as vulnerable as paid staff. Experience suggests that they may even be more vulnerable as their link with the hospice is more tenuous.

Volunteer support therefore is of prime importance from the moment a volunteer becomes involved within the hospice (see also Chapter 6 on the support of volunteers). This is a collective responsibility involving all members of staff and volunteer colleagues on a day-to-day basis. Effective support enables the volunteer to give of his/her best and reduces the turnover of volunteers.

Support comes in many forms both informal and formal and is especially important when a death occurs in the hospice. A breakdown of a possible support strategy for volunteers is outlined below.

Informal support

This involves:

- day-to-day contact and involvement with staff and fellow volunteers;
- regular 'open door' interaction with the VSM;
- informal meetings and opportunities for discussion and exchange of ideas.

Formal support

This involves:

- pairing of new volunteers with a more experienced buddy or mentor;
- preparation for their role and ongoing information about the hospice;
- volunteer support and development meetings as part of an integrated general training programme;
- specific skills training;
- review for new volunteers at end of induction period;
- supervision sessions (individual or in teams) for all volunteers;
- one-to-one supervision and group supervision for bereavement befrienders and volunteers involved with children;
- ongoing informal review;

- spiritual support;
- counselling service.

Volunteer retention

If an effective volunteer recruitment and selection process is coupled with good support and supervision, volunteer retention is high. It is important to both the families and to staff that there is not a constantly changing team of volunteers.

Many people come into the life of the affected child and his/her family either during frequent hospital visits or in the home. In the hospice, they also meet different staff and volunteers; and consequently seeing the same faces and getting to know them, is extremely important.

Continuity is also important to staff who invest time in training volunteers to become effective in their area of work. If there is a high turnover of volunteers, staff are continually training new volunteers. This can result in staff feeling that volunteers are more of a drain on their time than a valuable support. A volunteer who comes in regularly over a long period of time becomes very skilled in his/her role and is a great resource to the hospice.

Regular monitoring and review also has a key role to play in retaining volunteers.

Volunteer review and service monitoring

It is vital for the smooth running of the service that regular review and monitoring is carried out. Volunteer review may be undertaken on an informal basis through informal discussion and team meetings or on a formal basis similar to that of staff appraisal.

For service monitoring to be effective the VSM must 'walk the job', meeting volunteers and staff on a regular basis and getting a feel for how the service is being delivered and received. It is important to hear volunteers' views, ideas and suggestions and these should be built into future planning of the volunteer programme.

Dealing with difficult situations emerging from monitoring

If there is a spirit of trust and respect between people working together, the number of occasions when serious problems arise should be minimal. If they do, however, it is important that guidance exists on how to deal with the situation. Volunteers and staff should be aware of the procedure for dealing with difficulties.

There are usually a number of options[4] open to the VSM in dealing with difficulties with volunteers. These include:

- Retraining.
- Finding a different role.
- Asking the volunteer to take a break for a short time.
- Mentoring.

Except in serious cases, these options should be explored before deciding to dismiss the volunteer. It may be necessary in the last resort, however, to ask a volunteer to leave and this should be done sensitively and with honesty. Reasons which would prompt the dismissal of a volunteer include:

* Inappropriate behaviour towards the children or families.
* Theft, fraud.
* Continual breaching of guidelines.
* Breakdown of working relationships.
* Alcohol or substance abuse whilst on duty.

Training

Ongoing training is an important part of helping volunteers to maximize their skills and effectiveness (see also Chapter 5). It also assists in continuing to keep volunteers motivated. Increasingly, hospices are expected to ensure that volunteers in certain areas of work undertake 'statutory' training (e.g. food hygiene, moving, and handling).

For volunteers working with children it is vital that they undertake a preparatory course in addition to the induction programme. Topics might include: child protection, children's conditions, importance of play, communicating with children who cannot communicate, and issues and dilemmas in working with children and families.

Volunteer management in a children's hospice

The role of the Volunteer Service Manager (VSM) is not inconsiderable. He or she may be responsible for the greatest number of people in the organization, as in some hospices volunteers frequently outnumber paid staff. It is therefore important that an effective management system is in place to ensure the smooth running of the service and the effective supervision and support of volunteers. This management process involves:

* Design of volunteer roles and role descriptions.
* Recruitment and selection.
* Induction and training.
* Support and motivation of volunteers and staff involved with volunteers.
* Recognition of volunteers.
* Strategic planning and development of the service.
* Keeping statistics on volunteer activity.
* Keeping up-to-date personnel records.
* monitoring and evaluation.

The challenge of managing volunteers is that of managing a service on which the hospice depends. Given that this service is entirely made up people donating their leisure time and who are free to leave without any notice, effective rostering is vital to ensure continuity of service. This also allows volunteers to plan around their days at the hospice.

The VSM is frequently involved in managing a diverse age group of people ranging from children to the elderly. The skills and abilities of volunteers also cover a broad spectrum, including those who may require considerable support. The VSM therefore requires a clear understanding of the needs of the hospice and the issues involved, considerable people skills and the ability both to plan successfully and to deal quickly and effectively with crises.

Volunteer records

Each volunteer should have a personnel record. This ought to include copies of their application form, interview form, references, emergency contact details, and confirmation that a Criminal Records Office check has been carried out. This gives evidence that all stages of recruitment were completed. Records of training undertaken should also be kept in the file. Volunteer records should be accorded the same confidentiality as those of staff and volunteers should be able to see any information held about them.

Databases are valuable in holding volunteer information and allow speedy interrogation and retrieval. These need not be expensive as database software is available in computer packages and is more than adequate for the purpose. It is necessary however to comply with the terms of the Data Protection Act in keeping any information on volunteers whether paper or electronic (see Chapter 13 on legal issues).

Rotas/rosters

Volunteer Service Managers tend to have their own preferred way of timetabling volunteers. In some hospices, this may be carried out by the VSM or be devolved to the staff in each area or to experienced volunteers sometimes known as team organizers. Experience has shown that a system based on the principles of school timetabling is effective and economical of time. With this system, each day is divided into two or three sessions as required. Volunteers are asked to commit to the same day and time each week. Once recruitment has successfully filled all the sessions, the only work required in maintaining the rota is in finding cover for absent volunteers. This system obviates the need for making up weekly or monthly rotas and only requires revision when a volunteer leaves or changes his/her day.

Statistical information

It is invaluable, in fact essential, to keep statistics on the volunteer service. This helps with planning future services, shows trends in activity, and can be used for audit purposes and to demonstrate the significant work undertaken by volunteers. This may even help with matched funding applications. Information which is helpful to keep includes the:

- number of volunteers;
- age range;
- number volunteer visits to each area weekly, monthly and annually;
- number of volunteer hours worked in each area weekly, monthly and annually;
- training and meetings attended by volunteers;
- number of journeys undertaken by drivers;
- distances undertaken by drivers;
- number of volunteers who leave each year;
- ratio of staff to volunteers;
- economic value of voluntary service and the return on investment.

The challenges of volunteer involvement

Concern has been expressed from time to time that there are risks associated with involving volunteers in a children's hospice environment. If volunteers are effectively recruited, selected, inducted, supervised, and managed, there should be no more risks attached to volunteers than to paid staff. The key role for a Volunteer Service Manager is about minimizing risk.

Any problems which may be encountered are far outweighed by the benefits. Problems often occur not because people are volunteers, but because when any group of people work together difficulties may arise.

Boundaries

Often, when volunteers and staff work together there is the potential for difficulties arising from lack of understanding of each other's roles. Volunteers offering a service, such as complementary therapy, can engender professional rivalry or resentment from paid staff. This blurred boundary situation needs careful and sensitive management (see Chapter 14 on ethical issues).

Flexibility

The complete flexibility of the children's hospice environment can be difficult for some volunteers who have a need to be busy with an organized work schedule. For these people the area of work must be chosen very carefully and they are seldom successful at working with children. Volunteers are sometimes apprehensive initially about interacting with profoundly disabled children or bereaved families. Effective induction and training can help to prepare volunteers. The support and guidance of staff, however, is vital in helping them to develop skills and confidence in these areas.

Young volunteers

A children's hospice is all about children, young people, and their families. Young people aged between 16 and 21 have much to offer as volunteers. Hospices are often reluctant to involve this age group as they feel that they would need a great deal of support given their closeness in age to some of the affected children. A recent study demonstrated that these fears were unfounded.[5] Children's hospices which involved young volunteers found that with effective selection, support, preparation, and training, young volunteers can be a real asset to a children's hospice. The young people themselves reported that although initially anxious, they quickly settle. They cited the relaxed and friendly environment and the support of an older volunteer as being important.

Conclusion

The rewards from involving volunteers are significant. Their generosity of time and spirit is immense. They offer children and families another avenue for support and other ears to listen. Volunteers can be many things to many people: a young able-bodied companion for affected teenagers; a young 'friend' for siblings to interact with; a peer for mothers and fathers to relate to; an older parent figure to understand and support; an extra pair of hands to share the load with staff; an added source of laughter and fun and most importantly, another member of the children's hospice family.

Appendix 1
Children's Hospice Association Scotland (CHAS)*
Volunteer interview

Applicant's name:

Reasons for wanting to be a volunteer with CHAS:

What candidate hopes to gain from volunteering:

Current/previous work and voluntary experience:

What candidate enjoys doing and why:

Why children/experience of children:

Dealing with loss and bereavement (Rachel House and Children's Hospice Information Centre Only):

Health:

Availability:

Reaction to smoking policy:

Questions asked:

Explain next stage: ☐   Ask permission to approach referees: ☐

If driving for CHAS discuss:

Insurance: ☐   Driving licence: ☐   Drivers declaration: ☐

Decisions with reasons: YES/NO

Interviewers:_____   _____

Date: _____   _____

*Appendices 1 and 2 are reproduced by kind permission of the Children's Hospice Association of Scotland.

Appendix 2
Children's Hospice Association Scotland (CHAS)
Interview: volunteers working with children

1. What made you want to come forward to work with the children?

1b. What age groups do you prefer to work with?

2. What experience of children either in work or home like do you have which you feel will be helpful to you as a volunteer in this setting?

3. Discuss type of activities in which volunteers will be involved. How do you feel about this?

3b. What would you do if you found yourself with a group of five 4 to 12-year-olds and the Activities Co-ordinators were off ill?

4. What rights do you feel children have?

5. Whilst you are working as a volunteer you find a child behaving in a way that you personally find unacceptable. How would you handle this?

6. Any questions?

Explain about preparation day Trial period

Decisions with reasons:

Interviewers:_____   _____

Date: _____   _____

References

1. Association of Children's Hospices (ACH). *What is a children's hospice?* ACH, Bristol. Available from ACH, Kings House, 14 Orchard Street, Bristol, BS1 5EH, UK.
2. National Centre for Volunteering. *Screening volunteers.* www.volunteering.org.uk
3. Gold E (1997). The role and the need for the children's hospice in the United Kingdom. *International Journal of Palliative Nursing,* 3No(5), 281–6.
4. McCurley S and Lynch R (1998) *Essential volunteer management* (2nd edn), Directory of Social Change, London.
5. Scott R (2001). *Volunteering for the future—An evaluation of the effects on young volunteers of working in palliative care.* (In press - Hospice Bulletin)

Recommended reading

Dailey A and Zarbock Goltzer S (1993). *Hospice care for children.* Oxford University Press, New York.

Chapter 11

Volunteers working in a bereavement service

Do bereaved people need help and if so what intervention is helpful? What happens to the survivors when a person dies? No one person's reaction to loss is the same as another's but the pain of grief is universal and many of the experiences surrounding death and bereavement are universal. When planning a bereavement service these fundamental questions need to be addressed. Dr Colin Murray Parkes speaks of bereavement as having a detrimental effect upon physical and mental health.[1]

Help for the bereaved should be deeply rooted in the culture and community in which it is being experienced. In western society today, we avoid talking about death and we have largely abandoned the rituals with which our ancestors dealt with death. It is possible to reach adult life without ever having first-hand experience of death or a funeral. The sympathy of relatives and friends is all too often aimed at preventing rather than promoting the expression of grief so that open expression of pain and sadness is usually discouraged.

Different cultures have different ways of coping with grief; what is expected and considered normal in one culture is taboo in another. In some cultures, the whole community is involved but in others the families are left isolated and alone. In East Africa, for instance, death is seen as a natural part of life; people seldom die in hospital but on mats on the floor of their huts and the grief of the family is shared by the whole community.

Whatever our culture or society, the pain of bereavement needs to find appropriate expression. There is a universal need to talk about the death, to go over again and again the events associated with the loss, to accept it, and find a meaning to carry on with life. The bereaved need permission to grieve. Fortunately, most people do get through their grief with the support of their family and friends but for those who need help, hospices are in an ideal position to provide it. The question for the hospice or palliative care service is: 'Is there a need for a bereavement service?' and if one is operated, the question for the Bereavement Service Co-ordinator is: 'Where do I begin and who should be involved?'

No single approach

A bereavement service must be wanted. It must be designed to meet real, identified needs.[2] What are the needs of the bereaved? Befriending, counselling, support groups, practical help, social clubs, memorial services?

The list is a long one and will be influenced by the ethnic, cultural, and social groups to which people belong and whether any bereavement support already exists in their area. Personal research of the services provided by other British hospices showed that many different approaches were used with priority being given to opportunities for the bereaved to share their grief in a one-to-one relationship. In many cases, volunteers were being used to provide this support.

Research carried out by the Bereavement Care Standards UK Project estimated that 80% of bereavement support in Britain is delivered by the voluntary sector (that is to say, non-statutory, unpaid, and charity-funded) and 90% of it by volunteers.[3]

The successful placing of volunteers to support the terminally ill and their families in their own homes over many years led naturally to the decision to use volunteers as providers of bereavement care. It was important, however, to be clear about the role of the bereavement volunteers and what they are equipped and can be trained to do.[4]

Volunteers: a link to the community

Why are volunteers rather than professionals so widely involved in providing bereavement care in British hospices? If volunteers are drawn from a wide variety of backgrounds and life experiences they not only represent the community but provide a link to it. Volunteers demonstrate that bereavement is not a mental or physical illness but a normal reaction to the loss of someone close. 'The widespread involvement of volunteers underlines the concept that grief is natural. Volunteers are ordinary people and carry none of the stigma attached to mental health services, counselling or therapy'.[4]

Volunteers fulfil many different roles within the hospice and may continue to work in these areas in addition to supporting bereaved families. Their roles may include working on the wards, with the community volunteer team, in day care, or as a driver, hairdresser or lay chaplain. Volunteers working on the wards may develop the kind of supportive relationships that make them the best person to support a family member after bereavement.[5]

> A volunteer working on the ward shared with a family the powerlessness of watching the lingering death of father and husband. His wife struggled with her pain and distress at watching the suffering of her husband and confided to the volunteer that she did not think she could ever live without him. After he died she did not respond at first to offers of support feeling, as she told us 'that I have to put on a brave face'. Now, with her grief still raw and bubbling to the surface, she is responding well to help from the same volunteer who befriended her on the ward and who remembers her husband and all that he and the family suffered. She does not have to pretend any more.

Volunteers are unpaid but they are not amateurs! With careful selection, the right training, supervision, and support they are ideally placed to offer families bereavement support.

The selection minefield

Who makes a good bereavement volunteer and how do we recognize them? Unlike many other forms of voluntary work bereavement counselling rarely brings immediate satisfaction. We are asking volunteers often to visit someone they have not met before and to make this visit on their own. The family want their dead returned to them, and the effort of talking about their loss is exceedingly distressing and they may be reluctant to communicate.[2] Volunteers have to be able to stay with depression and pain through weeks or months without seeing much change or becoming too discouraged. They have to be comfortable with the sharing of painful feelings, tears, and anger. They have to be able to listen without giving advice.

Such people need to have sensitivity, warmth, common sense, courage, and realism. They must be good listeners, non-judgemental, and able to cope with the anxieties and fears of the bereaved. Bereavement counselling can sometimes reawaken the counsellor's own painful feelings of loss and volunteers need to be self-aware and accepting of supervision.

Experience has shown that trawling for new bereavement volunteers from amongst volunteers and staff who have already been working in other disciplines in the hospice for at least six months has many advantages. They have been exposed to the philosophy of palliative care and have had experience of working with death and dying before they apply to work with the bereaved. In addition to the interview process insights about the suitability of the applicant can be sought from the Voluntary Service Manager (VSM) or their line manager/team leader. This reduces the risk of selecting volunteers unsuited to the task and is an ideal method of recruitment if few volunteers are required, or are additions to an already established team. If larger numbers are needed it is unlikely that enough volunteers will come forward in-house to make this method of recruitment viable. In this case, recruitment will need to be on a much wider basis through advertisements in the community and word of mouth. A good method of recruitment is to offer a training course on loss and bereavement to the local community. This usually attracts many different people. At the end of the course any participants who are interested in becoming bereavement volunteers are invited to apply.

Many people are drawn to this type of work because of personal experience but not all are suitable. Some may unconsciously be searching for a way of working through their own grief or loss. It can sometimes be difficult to distinguish between potential helpers and those needing help for themselves. Doing this work often brings to the surface past losses or difficulties. If these have not been sufficiently resolved, training and supervision sessions risk becoming personal therapy for individual volunteers.[4] Unresolved grief can linger for many years and it is important to look for signs of continuing difficulties at interview.

The selection of bereavement volunteers needs to be as thorough as possible. It is not only the service but also the volunteers and their families who have to live with the stress and tension which can be caused by an unwise decision.[2] If there is any uncertainty as to suitability it is better to reject a volunteer than to take them on for this type of work. Mistakes can lead to a lack of confidence in the service by the bereaved and feelings of failure, anger, and disappointment in the volunteer.

The application form

Selection should be a two-way process enabling potential volunteers to find out what is involved in the role of helping bereaved people as well as enabling judgements to be made about their suitability. It is beneficial to invite those interested in volunteering to attend an informal discussion where they have the opportunity to meet with active volunteers, learn about what is involved and ask questions.

Those who decide to proceed should be given a simple application form to complete. The purpose of this form is to ask them to think about their motives for wanting to work with bereaved people and their understanding of what is involved.

Application forms should request information on:

- Name, address and telephone number.
- Date of birth.
- Current driving licence or any transport difficulties.
- Details of current occupation or hospice voluntary work.
- Any experience, training or qualifications relevant to working with bereaved people.
- Brief details, including dates, of any major personal loss including bereavement, redundancy, divorce or separation and serious illness.
- Name, address and telephone number of one or two referees who can vouch for their suitability for this type of work.
- Short (400 word) essay: 'What makes you interested in helping bereaved people? What is the role of a bereavement volunteer and what qualities and skills do you feel you have that would enable you to do this kind of work?'

The completed application form will enable a judgement to be made as to whether the applicant should be called forward for interview.

A two-tiered model for selection

A most effective method of selecting volunteers for bereavement work is to approach selection in two stages; an individual interview followed by a group case study. Applicants are usually nervous at interview and judgements made about their suitability may then be checked out as the case study progresses. It is helpful to have two interviewers as this enables a more objective and professional approach and allows a joint decision about the applicant to be made.

It is important to prepare for and structure the interviews to focus on:

- motivation for wanting to work with the bereaved;
- interests and beliefs;
- attitudes and prejudices;
- past losses and crises and how these were handled;
- how they support and sustain themselves;
- their own family;
- empathy, openness, and sensitivity;
- intelligence and willingness to learn;
- any relevant past experience;
- accepting of supervision;
- ability to work in a group.

Interviewers also need to be alert for non-verbal communication and any emotional undercurrents.

Following interview all applicants are then asked back to participate in a group case study. Cases and scenarios are presented to the group for discussion or alternatively the group is asked to take part in a 'sculpt', an experiential learning technique, if this technique is known. In either case, the attitudes, opinions, and skills of the applicants give the interviewers valuable insights as to their suitability for working with the bereaved.

Selection needs to be ongoing throughout initial training and the probationary period.

Which training course?

Volunteers bring with them the individual qualities for which they have been selected, their life experiences and their own tested ways of handling crises and disappointments. The challenge is how to train them without de-skilling them or devaluing the personal contributions that they bring.[2] Volunteers need initial preparation to work with the bereaved and ongoing training helps them to build and develop their skills. Initial training should cover:

- *Knowledge*—to acquire an understanding of loss and bereavement, theories and models of grief.
- *Skills*—practice in basic counselling skills.
- *Self-awareness*—awareness of how their own feelings and experiences may help or hinder the counselling process.

The course needs to be a balance of theory and practical with role-plays and experiential exercises so that theory is constantly demonstrated in practice. An average course will take 40–60 hours and may need to be run on an annual basis. A course of this nature is a huge commitment and can present difficulties with financial, time, and venue constraints. It is more easily achieved with larger numbers of participants who can benefit from the varied interests and experiences of the group. The experience of shared training with other bereavement agencies in the area can be useful and may build worthwhile bridges for the future. Some British hospices share training with Cruse Bereavement Care (a nationwide bereavement service in the UK staffed by volunteers) which cuts down on the workload and is beneficial to both organizations. Cruse has excellent trainers, hospices have good venues and support services, and the volunteers benefit from being with a large and varied group. At the end of the course the bereavement volunteers receive additional hospice sessions to cover the systems, paperwork, confidentiality, supervision, and other related issues particular to the hospice bereavement service. In Britain, an excellent initial training course has been produced by Cruse Bereavement Care UK and Help the Hospices with well-researched and evaluated sessions, handouts, and notes.[6]

Most volunteers find the commitment and sacrifice of giving up so much time to initial training well worth it. Some volunteers have described their experiences of initial training as 'life-changing', 'I find the skills work so well on my friends', 'I used to give advice but now I never do', 'my husband and I don't argue as much now'.

What's in a name?

The volunteers have completed their training and are ready to start their probation but what should they be called?

The advantage of using volunteers to support the bereaved is that they are not health care professionals but ordinary people. People who are grieving may know that they are not suffering mental or physical illness but a normal reaction to the loss of someone close. The word 'counsellor' may wrongly imply the need for therapeutic intervention or, alternatively, that the volunteer is trained to a higher level. It is important to choose a name for the team which gives the right message.

In recent years, there has been a debate in the Britain as to the use of the word 'counsellor' for those trained to work with grief. The truth is that bereavement often acts as a catalyst for the resurfacing of unresolved emotional difficulties from the past and over time many bereavement counsellors seek additional training, knowledge, and skills.

Volunteer teams in British hospice bereavement services are called by different names, amongst them 'bereavement support workers', 'bereavement visitors', 'befrienders', 'bereavement counsellors', and 'skilled helpers'. A group of newly trained volunteers who were asked what they wished to be called opted for 'bereavement volunteers' which they felt was a good compromise.

Unlike other hospice volunteers the identification badges of the bereavement volunteers do not give their surnames. They are known to their clients by their first names and may only be contacted through the Bereavement Service Co-ordinator. This is to protect them from unsolicited telephone calls or visits from bereaved people who often become distressed and lonely especially in the evenings and at weekends.

Launched: the probationary period

The volunteer is trained and ready to help their first bereaved person. It is important that they fully understand what is expected of them and what their boundaries are. Guidelines are issued to all bereavement volunteers along with their confidentiality document to sign. The guidelines set out the particular details of working within the bereavement service, what commitment is expected, supervision and support, any required paperwork regarding client visits, how to claim expenses, disciplinary and complaints procedures, and any other issues relevant to the service.

New bereavement volunteers are given one case to start with and after their first visit receive one-to-one supervision either by telephone or face-to-face. In addition to this they attend monthly supervision meetings in a group with other volunteers who have different levels of expertise. This is helpful for them to debrief on their feelings, usually of nervousness, their musings about whether the visit was helpful for the client and any difficulties. Affirmation and reassurance are extremely important. It is beneficial for the co-ordinator or supervisor to have an open door policy for bereavement volunteers to contact them about a client at any time. New volunteers will often wish to talk through each visit for the first few times until they become more confident and understand the usefulness of their monthly group supervision.

Probation normally lasts for six months but is dependent on the volunteer having sufficient exposure to clients during that period. The number of clients is not as important as the number of contacts. Probationers are treated in the same way as the other bereavement volunteers but their work is monitored more closely. They also attend ongoing training and team meetings. Probation is ended when both the supervisor and volunteer feel that the time is right. The selection process continues until the period of probation has ended.

It is important to allocate cases to probationers at the right skills level if possible. Beginners trying to help cases of abnormal grief or complicated family dynamics may feel unable to cope. Regular monthly supervision, preferably in small mixed-expertise groups, is vital for all bereavement volunteers.

The supervisor as 'enabler'

Volunteers who work with the bereaved need supervision. They need a safe forum where they are encouraged to explore their way of working with clients and look at any reawakened memories of personal losses or difficulties. The primary purpose of supervision is to provide support, ensure accountability, and that boundaries are being maintained, and to enhance and develop skills.[3] The initial training course together with any ongoing courses should cover the formal education responsibilities of the service. Supervisors fill in gaps on knowledge and make practical what was once 'head'-knowledge and must now become working-knowledge.[7] Supervision safeguards the wellbeing of the client, ensuring that his/her needs are being met and facilitates the professional and personal development of the volunteer. Volunteers will have uniquely different qualities, styles, and ways of working; the supervisor acts as an enabler for these gifts to be used to the best advantage with clients.

Supervision is achieved in a *small monthly mixed-expertise group* where the volunteers are exposed to a variety of different cases and styles of working. This supervision is mandatory with provision being made for holidays and illness. Easy access to the supervisor at other times is also essential, as has been stressed already, as volunteers may occasionally feel the need to talk if they are struggling with a difficult case or personal issues. In addition, they attend an individual annual supervision and work appraisal which gives them an opportunity to explore issues of personal development, ongoing training needs, and discuss any difficulties. Volunteers look forward to supervision and most say that they benefit from the time spent with their peers and find the case discussions interesting and helpful.

Supervisors should be counsellors experienced in working with loss and bereavement who have undertaken a course in how to supervise. It is also expected that the supervisor will also be supervised and their work and role be monitored.[3] Wherever possible, an external supervisor should be appointed. The question of who should supervise the bereavement volunteers may be governed by financial constraints so that the Bereavement Service Co-ordinator may fulfil this role along with the roles of trainer and manager of the service.

Volunteers working with clients

How many cases should a volunteer be given? Pressure of referrals to the service should never be passed on to the volunteers. The time that they are able to give to this work varies enormously according to their personal commitments. Volunteers are allocated one client and take on additional cases after discussion of complexity, frequency of visits, their own availability, and other considerations. Most volunteers handle two cases concurrently.

Bereavement services allocate cases in different ways. In some hospices, volunteers are the first people to have contact with the bereaved but this may present dangers in exposing volunteers to inappropriate referrals, complex cases or hazardous situations. If the client's first contact is with an experienced counsellor, nurse, or supervisor this can be avoided. The insights gained into a client's difficulties and past history provide invaluable assistance in the appropriate allocation of cases and allow complex cases to be handled by a more experienced counsellor. It also provides a vehicle for the filtering of inappropriate referrals where there may be a need to refer on to the psychological or psychiatric services or to the client's medical practitioner. Such invaluable information and insights are best provided by the 'care team' members in the hospice, nurses, doctors, social workers, and others who have cared for the patient, possibly both at home and in the hospice, and met many members of the family.

This first interview with the client, which may be at home or in the hospice, also gives an opportunity for their grief reaction to be 'normalized'. The strong emotions experienced in bereavement can prompt feelings of 'going mad' and when reassurance is given often no further support or intervention is necessary. The support offered by the service and the role of the bereavement volunteer is also explained enabling clients to make an informed choice about acceptance.

All are encouraged to return to the hospice to meet their bereavement befriender but there are many cases when this may not be possible or desirable and support is then given through home visits. Whether at hospice or home the frequency of visits is dependent on the degree of help needed. It is usual for visits to be more frequent at first with increasingly longer gaps as the client feels more able to cope. The number of visits is not set and the management of each case is monitored in supervision to ensure that the support given is enabling and empowering for the client and that dependency is not being created. Endings need to be managed sensitively and can be difficult for both the client and the bereavement volunteer.

Compassion fatigue

Folk wisdom tells us that when the waves crash in, no matter how hard the rock it will erode over time.[8]

Continually witnessing pain and grief can have a cumulative emotional impact which can make it difficult for volunteers to continue to offer support.[3] In some cases, the cause may be obvious and related to the particular bereavement they are supporting but in other cases it is less obvious. It may have nothing to do with their work but with outside events, home and family, friends, hospice staff or other volunteers. These can upset and interfere with the support systems they have come to rely on.[9] Such feelings may make a volunteer feel overwhelmed, insecure or ashamed. It is important that volunteers are offered emotional support in addition to supervision.

Time spent in supervision should centre on the work with the client. It may pick up emotional difficulties for a volunteer in handling a particular case but it is not the place to give attention to the needs of volunteers in fulfilling this role. An open door policy for support is important as well as keeping a watchful eye on the team in an attempt to avoid casualties. Caring for each other and peer support is also encouraged. It is sometimes, but not always, possible to predict when problems may occur. Emotional involvement and over-identification with clients, feelings of anger, spiritual distress, depression, unusual sensitivity or irritability are all signs that something may be amiss. In such instances, volunteers are given the opportunity for confidential counselling and support from the staff support counsellor appointed from an outside agency. There is no stigma attached to 'resting' from bereavement work for a while. A few volunteers take time-out during a personal crisis or difficulty such as illness and family difficulties. A gentle easing back into casework is facilitated when the volunteer feels ready.

The support offered by the hospice will only be useful if volunteers take on the responsibility of caring for themselves and are aware of their own weaknesses and vulnerabilities. It is also important to foster a good team spirit with opportunities for humour and a pervading sense of hope. The occasional social event provides an ideal opportunity for this.

Safety: whose responsibility is it?

A difficult bereavement visit was a forceful reminder of the importance of having a safety policy in place for home visits. The house was in an isolated spot, the bereaved gentleman appeared very strange and was accompanied by an evil-tempered dog. It soon became apparent that discussing his bereavement was the least of his intentions. Extrication was difficult and frightening.

Inclusion of discussion on issues of personal safety, potential dangers, and common sense practical guidelines should form part of the volunteer's initial training course, with reminders annually. Hospices need to take all reasonable precautions to ensure the safety of their volunteers but responsibility for personal safety has to ultimately rest with the person making the visit.

Guidelines on safety for volunteers

- The volunteer should always let family or hospice know where they intend to go.
- The volunteer should let family or hospice know the expected duration of the visit.
- The volunteer must remember to advise the hospice if plans are altered.
- Safety guidelines must be issued to all bereavement volunteers, highlighting the importance of trusting their instincts and judgements and using their common sense. Volunteers should never feel pressurized into making a home visit if they have any doubts, and if they feel uncomfortable in any situation they should make an excuse and leave immediately.
- Volunteers should be asked to report any incidents, however small, to the hospice. Training needs to include skills in the diffusion of anger and threatening behaviour.

Ongoing training

The initial training course gives the volunteer the essential basic knowledge and skills to work with bereaved people. Practical experience of working with different clients, supervision, and ongoing training will increase these skills. Needs for additional training are identified by both the supervisor and the volunteers who are encouraged to identify their own gaps in knowledge and skills. Opportunities are given for volunteers to research and present topics of interest to share with their peers. Case studies, role-plays, brainstorming, videos, experiential exercises, and 'sculpting' are all used. Sculpting is a particularly helpful technique used to provide insights into relationships, alliances, and feelings in family or group dynamics. Involvement and participation by the volunteers increases their knowledge of theories, their self-awareness, and confidence. Ongoing training is done in-house on a quarterly basis when the whole team have an opportunity to get together. It is combined with a brief administrative period when hospice and issues pertaining to the bereavement service and volunteers are dealt with. These quarterly meetings also foster a team spirit by providing a regular opportunity for sharing and peer support.

Volunteers are also encouraged to read and provide items of interest for circulation from newspaper or magazine articles, book or film reviews.

Hospice bereavement care: a proactive approach

Unlike many other agencies in the community, hospices have the opportunity to be proactive in offering help, support, and information to the bereaved. We do not have to wait until problems occur to give help. It is important to keep a balance between offering initial support and making a family feel that they are unable to cope. All bereaved families are given the opportunity of a routine visit six weeks to two months following the death. This visit is then made by the Bereavement Service Co-ordinator who is able to make an assessment of needs. Allocation to a volunteer in then made if further help is requested at this stage. Bereaved people who are considered more at risk or vulnerable are targeted earlier through a well-researched bereavement profile questionnaire. This gives details of the death, the family relationships, known social support networks, and other predisposing factors.[10] It is completed, as has been explained above, by the multidisciplinary care team and discussed at the weekly ward clinical meeting with the Bereavement Service Co-ordinator who is able to make an assessment of risk. Any one who has been identified as at risk of having difficulties are offered support at an earlier stage through a telephone call by a volunteer.

Hospice bereavement care is offered within the context of palliative care. The nursing and pastoral care teams who care for families in the period leading up to the death often know them well. At this time, the needs of the patient take precedence and relatives will often deny their own feelings of grief in order to keep control and continue to care for the dying person.[5] Involvement of the bereavement service is only requested if complex issues, such as multiple prior bereavements, are identified. Bereavement volunteers will give in-depth support to these family members and occasionally to patients who are anticipating and grieving their own deaths. In such cases, the volunteers receive additional one-to-one supervision.

Once the death has occurred, the bereaved family are referred to the bereavement service for ongoing support. All families are offered two opportunities to attend bereavement afternoons or evenings staffed by a team of nurses and volunteers. The aim of these events is to give an opportunity for families to return to the hospice, to 'normalize' grief, and to enable bereaved people to meet each other.

Volunteers who are not bereavement volunteers, help at these events by welcoming families back to the hospice, serving refreshments and making them feel at home. They are not regarded as bereavement counsellors but are given training in listening skills and basic theories of loss and bereavement. Because families usually like to see the nurses who cared for their loved ones and helped the relatives at the time of the death some nurses also attend. Such events offer an opportunity to meet and share with other people who have been bereaved in a welcoming environment with which they are familiar. However, as has been noted, not everyone wants to go back to the hospice.

Help for bereaved children

Many British hospices help bereaved children by offering a service especially tailored to their needs. Some have appointed separate co-ordinators for adult and children's bereavement services. Many of the children's services also help bereaved children in the local community and are run jointly with community services. Children benefit greatly by meeting other children who are bereaved and group work is often offered in preference to individual counselling.

Surviving parents, families, close friends or teachers with whom the child has a good relationship are usually the best people to support grieving children. Information on how children grieve and support for families before and after the death are offered but there are some occasions when children need individual support. Volunteers working with children should have experience working with bereaved adults before undertaking additional training. This training needs to cover the way children and adolescents grieve, creative ways of working with children, and resources that can be used. Criminal record checks are necessary under the UK Child Protection Act for any team member who offers one-to-one support to children.

The hospice bereavement service: a community resource

The hospice bereavement service is a resource for the community offering information about grief, education, and training to professionals and workshops to community and faith groups. Volunteers play a large part in 'normalizing' the process of grieving in the community and in helping society to see that there is a need to support those who are suffering after the death of someone close.

Bereavement volunteers: the last word

The last word must come from the bereavement volunteers themselves. They admit that the going is often hard at times but the reward of seeing someone eventually move on with their lives cannot be measured. They say that they mostly 'enjoy' their work but comment that they are not sure that 'enjoy' is quite the right word!

References

1. Parkes CM (1991). *Bereavement: Studies of grief in adult life* (2nd edn). Penguin, London.
2. Earnshaw-Smith E and Yorkstone P (1986). *Setting up and running a bereavement service*. St. Christopher's Hospice, London.
3. *Standards for bereavement care in the UK* (2001). Bereavement Care Standards: UK Project. (Available from London Bereavement Network, 356 Holloway Road, London N7 6PA; also at: www.bereavement.org.uk)

4. Relf M (1998). Involving volunteers in bereavement counselling. *European Journal of Palliative Care,* **5**(2), 61–5.
5. Parkes CM (1998). Bereavement. In *Oxford Textbook of palliative medicine,* (ed. D Doyle, GW Hanks, and N MacDonald). Oxford University Press.
6. Faulkner A and Wallbank S (1998). *Bereavement counselling.* Help the Hospices and Cruse Bereavement Care. (Available from Help the Hospices 34–44 Britannia Street, London, WC1X 9JG.)
7. Carroll M (1996). *Counselling supervision.* Cassell, London.
8. Bowman T (1999). Promoting resiliency in those who do bereavement work. *Lifeline, Journal of the National Association of Bereavement Services,* **27**, Spring.
9. Parkes CM (1986). The caregivers griefs. *Journal of Palliative Care,* **1**(2); 5–6.
10. Parkes CM (1990). Risk factors in bereavement: Implications for the prevention and treatment of pathological grief. *Psychiatric Annals,* **20**(6), 310.

Recommended reading

Jeffrey D (2002). *Teaching palliative care, a practical guide.* Radcliffe Medical Press Abingdon.

Walshe C (1997). Whom to help? An exploration of the assessment of grief. *International Journal of Palliative Nursing,* **3**(3), 132–7.

Faulkner A (1998). *Working with bereaved people.* Harcourt Brace, London.

Chapter 12

Professionals working as volunteers

Very little has been published about the issues surrounding professionals who wish to contribute their professional skills as volunteers in a hospice/palliative care service—their selection, training, supervision, accountability, and the many planning issues that inevitably arise. It is important to avoid wasting the time of volunteers, as there is nothing as a rule that they hate more, and this is even more true of professional volunteers. But this is exactly what happens if there has been insufficient planning and vision to define and prepare for the work to be done.

This chapter will examine some of the factors that affect the integration of professional volunteers in a palliative care unit.

Why have professional volunteers?

Volunteering appears to be going through some changes related to the style in which people choose to participate. We are moving towards a system in which there are two distinct types of volunteers: (1) the long-term volunteer, who lives locally and has been trained in-house to provide a specific support task, and (2) the specialist volunteer bringing externally acquired expertise in to a hospice.

Specialist volunteering is gaining a higher profile with more people becoming aware of the option of donating not just their time, but a specific skill. This coincides with recent economic trends, which have heightened the commitment of palliative care units to make volunteering more effective.

As the definition and use of the word 'volunteer' changes, let us start by defining what we mean when we talk about professional volunteers in palliative care. This is a person that donates his/her specialist skills and time for a charitable purpose, mostly, although not exclusively to enhance the quality of physical care that is provided for patients.

The main reason why professional volunteers are such an asset in palliative care is because they donate their time and skills cost-free. They are obviously saving resources but crucially help a palliative care unit to provide additional skills and services that could not be funded out of the core budget.

Using volunteers that are highly skilled, often in an area that is not economically viable to attract funding gives unique opportunities to extend the quality and range of care that can be offered to patients and relatives. It makes it possible, for example, to introduce a new therapy that has not yet been evaluated to improve quality of life, but which may well establish itself as a core service in the future.

In what way are volunteers donating a professional skill different?

All the management principles that work effectively with volunteers apply to professional volunteers as well, but some of the common problems with volunteer involvement are thrown into sharper focus with professional placements.

These volunteers are likely to have a high expectation of being managed well, because they compare how their skill is valued in the marketplace. They are often highly skilled and are motivated to improve their skills in a specialist setting and have a good understanding of the value of their skill to the voluntary sector. This in turn leads to expectations to have an equal relationship with paid professional staff and have their opinions heard and acted on. They are confident in their approach and expect to have a certain amount of influence in the organizational decision-making process.

There is a growing trend to professionalize volunteer involvement and management. There are now different expectations from the senior management team in a palliative care unit about volunteer involvement, which coincide with changes in the economic climate. Palliative care units are constantly undergoing financial reviews, which has led to re-evaluating the workings of the multidisciplinary team. Professional volunteers as part of the team now not only complement but also extend core services.

We are also more inclined to follow the examples of some of the large-scale volunteer programmes found in the USA. There is a much greater emphasis on realizing the cost–benefit relationship of volunteering and measuring the value of donated time to a charity, which is then offset against project funding.

What kind of professional volunteer can be utilized?

There is potentially an endless list of people than can be involved and the variety of professionals on the team will be a combination of the vision of potential by the unit, of who applies, who is recruited and who is successfully integrated and stays. Some examples, but by no means an exclusive list are: health care workers, counsellors, physiotherapists, interpreters, receptionists, art and music therapists, hairdressers, beauticians. There is another, in most cases smaller, group of professional volunteers who work in non-patient care roles: for example, accountants, secretaries, and librarians.

For some professionals the motivation to donate their skills is similar to any volunteers. But for others it gives the opportunity to gain new experiences, develop, update their skills, and utilize them in a different context.

Recent trends suggest that there is a decline in the number of traditional 'not professionally educated and trained' female middle class volunteers who used to be the mainstay of additional help in a palliative care unit. Women are still more than three times as likely as men to be involved in volunteer activity, especially in health and social welfare work. They are also more likely to be involved in direct patient care than are men. Some of the changes in our society mean that more well-educated women now often have a professional career and balance this with family life. This means that a larger group of women *with professional skills* is now available, wishing to donate time to a charity *in their professional capacity.*

Complementary therapy is one of the areas were where professional volunteer services are increasing. Whilst this service has enhanced care and is clearly popular with patients, it has led to the new need to promote safe good practice in their clinical management.

Palliative care units are also seeing an increase in employee volunteering and secondments. Practice varies, but a typical employee volunteer will donate his professional skill for a few hours a month where it is needed, perhaps research a specific project or sit on a committee. Secondments are short- to medium-term placements often to assist in aspects of strategic planning and management.

Another demographic trend points to an increasingly older population who may retire early. This means not only will there be a greater need for services for older people, but crucially that there will be a larger pool of active volunteers to draw on. These retired professionals can be recruited for an unpaid or 'expenses only' second career.

Whatever the ultimate aims are for professional volunteer involvement, it is good management practice to start small. It makes sense to pilot new procedures and deal with problems that will only surface once a new placement has been introduced.

Case study: Introducing a new therapy.

Katie is a qualified Reiki healer who has worked with patients for the last ten years. She has her own thriving private practice and works from home, but she is keen to donate some of her time and skills to cancer patients. She is affiliated to the World Federation of Healing, which provides her with access to specialist insurance and support.

The concept of healing in working with patients who are suffering from life-threatening conditions or terminally ill patients has always been controversial, with the unspoken assumption that it raises false hopes of a cure. But as awareness of complementary therapies has become greater in the general population, the idea does get mentioned both by patients and potential volunteers who offer to provide this service. In this circumstance, the word 'healing' takes on a somewhat different meaning, emphasizing a return to greater wholeness, relaxation, and wellbeing. After the interview and verification of Katie's qualifications, references, and experience, Reiki as a speciality was discussed with the multidisciplinary team. As the demand for this therapy was patient-led a trial placement was agreed.

Case study (*continued*)

Utilizing Katie's professional skills gave patients access to another therapy, which would not have been funded by a palliative care provider. Through Katie's teaching and feedback from patients, staff were able to understand more about Reiki and its value for patients. The staff had to learn to manage a professional volunteer and reassess how they work as a team.

Issues arose about access to patient information, referral forms, job title, working space, and involvement in multidisciplinary meetings. All of these issues had to be resolved as a team and many are ongoing.

Reiki remains a popular therapy in the unit but is considered to be a controversial concept by many professionals.

This is an example of how a professional volunteer can be integrated into a team to offer a service that is not considered to be mainstream but one that more and more patients in a palliative care setting demand.

The application process

The most important step in deciding whether a professional volunteer will fit the team is by meeting face-to-face. This should precede written documentation and a formal interview. From a visit you can start to see an individual's personality and form an opinion whether someone will integrate into an existing team. It will be possible to pick up on what is motivating the potential applicant and what they expect from the palliative care unit. It may be that after an informal visit the volunteer decides not to apply, perhaps the unit does not meet his/her needs. If this is the case, then the visit has been of value as it has saved you and them a great deal of time. It is important that the applicants at this stage read the volunteer policy, which should detail their responsibilities. If they are not happy with the policy then there is little point in continuing with the application process.

Recruiting professional volunteers involves devising an appropriate, comprehensive application form, which supplies details a palliative care unit must have before accepting a professional volunteer.

It is crucial to know:

+ Qualifications.
+ Professional background.
+ Colleges/Schools.
+ Insurance.
+ Their motivations and expectations.

Ask about colleges, as some have a better reputation than others do and get information on the content of courses such as:

+ How long is the course?
+ Does it involve client contact?

- What is required before enrolment?
- What qualification do people graduate with?

The references taken up should be from someone who can comment on the professional's practice. If the applicant is a therapist then, ideally, one of the references should be from a former tutor. This information gives a good idea of how the professional works and whether his/her style of working will fit the unit.

It is important to check your organization's insurance policy as to whether specialist volunteer work is covered. If it is a volunteer complementary therapist they are likely to be affiliated to a professional body and have the option to take out personal insurance which may cover them whilst volunteering. Copies of the insurance policy must be kept on the volunteer file and updated annually (see also Chapter 13 on legal issues).

It is worth remembering that an established team has its own dynamics. A new recruit with a different style of working, especially if they introduce a new treatment, can cause major upheaval.

Ensure that the team understands what motivates a particular professional and assess whether the palliative care team can offer that experience. Specialist volunteers need support, supervision and training. In many ways, this is no different to what all volunteers need. However, a professional qualification may need updating and this has a cost implication. These costs need be considered before the volunteer is recruited.

An application process does not only consist of a completed application form but should involve an interview that will not just request but more crucially receive information from the professional volunteer. A volunteer with a speciality in a particular area will be a valuable addition to the service that is provided but will make greater demands on staff's time and resources.

Relations between paid and unpaid staff

The working relationships between staff teams are without doubt the most important factor in determining the success of professional placements. There are a number of reasons why paid staff might feel threatened by professional volunteers or in turn volunteers may be resistant to work well with employees.

Sometimes, paid staff assume that if someone works without payment he/she cannot be very good at what he/she does, while assuming that another paid member of the team is competent unless it is proven otherwise. The 'I am only a volunteer' syndrome is unhelpful. Volunteers must have feedback that they are an essential and valued part of the team. This also means giving unpaid members of staff a title and name badge that reflects the job they do

Volunteers should be invited by name to relevant team meetings. Their professional opinions should be listened to and they must be involved in planning decisions that affect their work. If volunteers are not involved in the planning and decision-making process and acquire a sense of ownership of their projects and patients, their motivation and pride of their achievements will diminish. Also, if there is lack of consistency in their management, different supervising staff working to different rules, this will mean that volunteers become confused, resentful, and powerless. This is especially true of volunteers that only work infrequent shifts.

If volunteers are highly trained in the skill they are donating, they can be a threat to inexperienced staff, with the implication that they might be difficult to manage. This can be avoided through effective two-way communication. As a member of the team, a professional volunteer can be is an equal member of the team and can be an effective educator to other staff.

Any one who works or volunteers in health care settings knows the importance of confidentiality. It is curious assumption that unpaid professional staff cannot be trusted with confidential information, and are more likely to be indiscreet. This attitude will be extremely divisive, as professional volunteers are no more likely to discuss their work than any other staff. Signing an agreement, appropriate training, and generating a forum for discussions will go some way towards reducing concerns. All paid and unpaid staff should work in an environment in which they have access to the information they 'need to know' to do their job. There should be no distinction for volunteers.

Supervision

The effectiveness of any volunteer programme is dependent on the quality of supervision volunteers receive. To ensure that professional volunteers can work effectively it is necessary to concentrate on building relationships that respect and recognize the competency and professionalism of all staff in the multidisciplinary team. Who is the best line manager to evaluate a speciality? It may take some serious consideration to find the most appropriate person to comment on another's clinical or nonclinical work. Careful thought should be given to the whole idea of supervision. If it cannot be provided internally there will be a cost implication.

Accountability

In the case of volunteers trained and working as health care professionals (doctor, nurse, physiotherapist, etc.) they should logically be accountable to their clinical line manager. The doctor is accountable to the senior doctor, the nurse to the senior nurse, and so on. What is not so obvious and therefore requires careful thought and planning before the volunteer starts work, is to whom a complementary therapist is accountable, a librarian, a computer specialist, a hairdresser or beautician. Whatever is decided must be explained to the volunteers before they start their work.

Grievances and discipline

Professional volunteers should be treated no differently to paid staff when it comes to grievances or disciplinary issues. This is why it is important to have a job description for each placement, which defines expectations of the standard and quality of the work expected. If there is a suggestion that a professional volunteer is not performing or adhering to policies or procedures, the organization's disciplinary procedure should be put into action. The fact that a professional works unpaid may lead supervising staff to be more lenient in dealing with performance issues, which should not be the case. This also applies to reviews or appraisals. Any professional will expect constructive feedback on their work.

Case study: Paid and volunteer nurses working in the same team.

Norman is a registered nurse who has recently retired early due to a minor medical problem. He loves being with patients and enjoyed a successful career in a large teaching hospital. When he approached his local palliative care unit he found that using volunteer nurses had not been considered. He was recruited as a general volunteer on the wards, talking to patients, making tea and coffee and various other volunteer duties. It soon became obvious that Norman had a lot more to offer and he expanded his role slowly. He helped to make beds, wash and shave patients, and assisted the nurses, as they required. The extra help was generally welcomed, but some staff were concerned that his extended role was not part, and should not be part, of what volunteers should do. Some nurses were also concerned about how using unpaid staff might affect their jobs. As in many hospices, the unit was undergoing changes and cutbacks had been made. Serious issues were raised like insurance cover, access to confidential notes, and meetings. The staff were concerned for Norman's safety and highlighted potential problem areas including manual handling, risk assessment, and infection control.

Further discussions with staff generated greater insight into their views on working with professional volunteers. It was made clear that volunteer nurses would always be additional to accepted staffing levels, and would be able to take some pressure off the rest of the team, but would never substitute for paid staff. The staff, in this case, were not happy for Norman to attend their team meetings to discuss, plan, and evaluate care they felt he was not therefore fully aware of issues surrounding patient needs.

The role of the volunteer in a nursing capacity that is an equal member of the nursing teams is one that this unit is not ready for. It would not be helpful to continue to advocate this type of nursing placement until the staff and management are fully supportive and keen to make it work.

A compromise was reached where Norman can make good use of his experience and skills without being subjected to the same pressures as the nursing staff.

Funding and facilities

When involving volunteers it is important to examine carefully the implications of having new members on the team. This is especially true when recruiting professional staff. They will expect the appropriate facilities and funding for the work they are proposing to do. Important considerations are access to desks and computers, availability of treatment rooms for therapists, lockers and changing rooms, uniforms, aprons or other protective clothing. Also, the cost of paying for equipment can be very high, depending on the skill being offered. If you are planning to recruit a hairdresser, you might well find they expect some of the equipment they are accustomed to in their working life outside the organization. Think about height-adjustable chairs, sinks, large mirrors, and pleasant surroundings. Consider whether the patients pay a contribution to this, often very popular, service or whether it will be offered without charge.

Another often forgotten cost is the option to contribute to the insurance cover for therapists, especially if they are newly qualified and do not have their own practice. By far the largest underestimated resource implication is the hidden cost of the management, support, and supervision of professional volunteers. To make the service work, volunteers need to have induction, on the job training, briefing and debriefing, and time for support sessions. Multiply this by the number of volunteers and then add the turnover. Further allow for the fact that they do about one shift per week and hence have different communication and update needs than full-time staff. You arrive at a substantial number of hours.

Is volunteer management included in paid staff job descriptions and if not will the staff find the time to look after the professional volunteers allocated to their department? Ward managers may feel that volunteers drain staff time from their real work. Specialist volunteers do need access to a supervisor. If a member of permanent staff finds that their manager is busy, the question can probably wait a while. But a volunteer may only be in the unit once a week. In that situation, a huge amount of time and, by implication, money is wasted if the volunteer cannot get on with their designated work.

Writing a policy about involving professional volunteers

Policy—a constitution, a course of action or an adapted and proposed principle. (Concise Oxford Dictionary)

Any written policy is a guideline and a useful tool to guide good practice. When writing a policy collectively you gain a consensus of opinion, thus facilitating an optimal volunteer environment, which ensures that paid and unpaid staff work together with clear goals and expectations.

The starting point for working with professional volunteers is in some ways no different than working with volunteers who have no specialist skills or training. Identifying where help is required, defining what that help is, highlighting the skills required, and evaluating the success of the project or placement remains crucial to any successful volunteer initiative. However, when working with professional volunteers there are a number of other key factors that need to be given careful consideration. These include:

♦ Volunteer expectations from volunteering.

♦ Staff ideas and reservations about working with an unpaid professional.

- Boundaries and frameworks within which the volunteer operates.
- Confidentiality and clinical information sharing.

It is hard to look at these issues when the volunteer is already working. It is far better practice to define key responsibilities before the volunteer commences his/her placement. The easiest way to do that is to write a policy.

Who should write the policy and who is it for?

It is best to have a group of people involved in a project like this. This way you will have a comprehensive, objective document. It is important to have a chairperson and someone to take detailed minutes. Policies should be working documents and are therefore subject to regular review by the policy writers. Depending on the size of the organization, a number of senior members of staff should be included to discuss strategic issues and certainly some representatives from the professions in question. The policy should be written to define key responsibilities, so that the paid and unpaid staff working together knows exactly what is expected of them.

What will be the content of the policy?

Included in the policy document should be the following:

- The title.
- The policy statement defining what we aim to achieve.
- The purpose.
- Definitions of the professions in question.
- The referral system.
- Patient consent and confidentiality.
- The responsibility of the volunteer, paid staff, and line manager.
- Criteria for accepting a volunteer in a professional capacity, including qualifications and experience required.

Consider the issue that although professionals may want to help, they will probably also want to expand their own paid private work. Is it acceptable to use the palliative care unit to make new contacts? What of the patient who is being discharged home but who wants to continue receiving the volunteer's aromatherapy or reflexology? The whole issue of the professional volunteer's boundary needs to be discussed and addressed *before* placement starts.

Conclusion

This chapter has highlighted some of the issues that need to be considered when using volunteers in palliative care, working in a professional capacity. It presents the challenge to utilize donated time and skills to the maximum, because volunteers cannot fully and successfully contribute to a hospice unless they are recognized and planned for by the management and staff. This points to certain dilemmas and each unit needs to weigh up the costs and benefits involved and decide how they would cope. Does the palliative care unit have the staff resources and commitments to supervise professional volunteers? These are key issues.

Key issues: Considerations when planning volunteer placements

- Have a job description in place for the placements you wish to recruit for.
- Identify line management responsibilities for professional roles.
- Ensure appropriate funding and facilities.
- Consider support and supervision needs.
- Write a policy.
- Training on confidentiality.
- Incorporate volunteer management issues in staff training.

Volunteering trends point to the fact that volunteering is becoming more professional, and expectations and standards are becoming more defined. The role of the Volunteer Services Manager has been extended to plan ahead, evaluate, and anticipate potential concerns. This is a change from the traditional role of direct volunteer supervision. Teaching staff about the management of professional volunteers has become a major aspect of the VSM's role.

A final thought. People are an organization's greatest asset and professional volunteers can potentially bring great benefits to service provision. The question is not whether volunteers can fill gaps in the budget, but whether a palliative care unit is truly prepared to utilize volunteers in teamwork with paid staff. The notion that professional volunteers offer a 'free service' remains one of the greatest challenges in planning for volunteer involvement.

Chapter 13

Legal issues for the Volunteer Service Manager

Palliative care services, in whatever country they operate, whether they are independent hospices or units attached to general hospitals, must be aware of their legal obligations to protect their employees, volunteers, patients, relatives, and the public. The Management Committee, Board of Trustees or Board of Directors—whatever is the title given to the governing body—has ultimate responsibility to ensure that these legal obligations are met.

If the Volunteer Service Manager (VSM) is paid, he/she is regarded as an *employee* of the organization, and, as such, should be protected by the Employment Laws of that country. If unpaid they will be considered as a member of the voluntary staff and, with the volunteers for whom the VSM is responsible, and who are also unpaid, will not be protected by Employment Law. In essence, voluntary staff/unpaid workers in any organization are protected by the laws which are in place for the protection of the general public.

General principles relevant to all working within a palliative care service

In order for the organization to exercise properly due care for all concerned—both paid staff and unpaid volunteers—certain steps should be taken. These *are not legally binding* but should include:

- All information and advice given by the organization should be accurate and up-to-date.
- All employees and volunteers who give information and advice should be properly trained, inducted, and supervised.
- Proper records should be kept of all information and advice given.
- Employees and volunteers should not be allowed to operate on their own with children or vulnerable adults, or be in situations where they have access to money or valuables until the organization has taken up references and has satisfied itself that the person in trustworthy.

- The premises and equipment should be safe and adequate training given in their use.
- There should be a clear and workable complaints procedure and all complaints should be seen to be taken seriously and properly investigated.

If those steps are not taken and there is a resulting injury or suffering to anyone connected with the organization or its clients, then the members of the governing body or its appointees could be sued for negligence. The range of insurance policies available to cover such situations are discussed below under the heading *Insurance policies.*

Checklist of relevant legislation

The duty of care applies to all organizations and individuals, whether paid or unpaid. It is essential that the items discussed below are considered carefully and put in place for the protection of employees and volunteers alike, although this chapter is concerned with volunteers only.

- Health and Safety Policy (see Appendix 1).
- Insurance Policies.
- Equal Opportunities Policy.
- Human Rights Act.
- Rehabilitation of Offenders Act.
- Police Act.
- Foreign nationals as volunteers.
- Asylum and Immigration Act.
- Data Protection Acts.

This chapter is written from a United Kingdom perspective. It is recognized that not all countries have the same legislation or safeguards, although many are very similar. Readers are advised to ascertain which laws and legal safeguards apply in their country and to ensure that they are implemented with regard to any volunteer service, however small it is.

Financial matters

Paid members of staff and volunteers

As mentioned already it is vital to recognize and understand the difference between a 'volunteer' and an 'employee'. It is more than simply one being paid and the other unpaid, or that Employment Law affects the paid member of staff and not the unpaid one. Their legal status, and tax liability, depend on the nature of any money transfer between the palliative care service and the volunteer, as explained below.

Another distinction between employee and volunteer is the number of hours involved in the duty undertaken. Most volunteers will commit to a few hours per week or one whole day per week. Paid staff usually work at least 16 hours per week if part-time, or more if a full-time employee. These working hours will vary from place to place. When volunteers receive payment in kind, such as training, care must be taken not to provide more than is absolutely necessary for the task. This can otherwise be construed as payment above the limit for their voluntary duty and so the volunteer could be considered to be in a contractual arrangement and so lose voluntary status.

◆ *Reimbursement.* This is the repayment for genuine, verifiable out-of-pocket expenses. This payment is not taxable and does not create a contractual or employment relationship. It will not affect state benefits (UK).

◆ *Earnings.* This is payment given in return for work. This remuneration is taxable, may create a contractual or employment relationship and may affect some state benefits (UK).

◆ *Other payments.* Under this heading might come such things as honoraria given to a volunteer who helps to manage a charity shop for the organization and 'session fees' paid to a complementary therapist.

These payments are not reimbursement, and may or may not be considered in law to be remuneration. They are likely to be taxable as 'earnings' and may in some situations create a contractual or employment relationship, and may affect state benefits.

The advice of a legal or tax expert should be sought if the Volunteer Service Manager has any doubts about these issues.

Expenses claim form1

Volunteers who are eligible for out-of-pocket reimbursement relating to a genuine expense to enable them to carry out their duty should always produce evidence, such as receipts and other relevant documents, and/or sign a claim form.[1] This will help the Inland Revenue/Tax Office to be convinced that the expenditure was actually incurred, was specific to the voluntary work, and necessary for the work to be carried out.

The claim forms should be clearly set out with the:

◆ volunteer's name;

◆ date of expenditure;

◆ nature of the expenditure;

◆ the reason for it; and

◆ the amount.

There should be space for the signature of the volunteer, date and cheque number, and signature of person authorizing the reimbursement. Evidence supporting the claim should be attached to the claim form.

Volunteer drivers

These are a special group. It is desirable that the VSM sees the driver's personal driving licence each year and when taking on a new driver has sight of the appropriate roadworthy certificate (in the UK, the Ministry of Transport Road Worthiness Certificate—MOT) and the car insurance certificate. Car and personal insurance are dealt with later in this chapter.

Those who use their own cars to bring patients into the hospice should have their mileage reimbursed. This will require a special claim form. In addition to the claimant's name it should ask the engine capacity of the car, the starting point and the end point of each journey on the speedometer, as well as total number of miles/kilometres claimed. Different countries will have their own rules for this but in countries, such as the UK, there is a tax implication. The total paid to a volunteer in any one year might exceed that allowed by the Tax Office, particularly when many miles/kilometres have to be travelled transporting patients in rural areas. Some units pay an arbitrary flat rate per mile/kilometre. It is, however, advisable to reimburse mileage at a nationally accepted rate, information about which can be found in the UK through the Inland Revenue PAYE enquiry office, the motoring organizations, and other national voluntary organizations. Similar motoring organizations exist in every country where palliative cares services operate

It follows that volunteer drivers must keep proper distance records. The VSM or someone delegated by him/her should check these. Tax Offices will have local information regarding this important reimbursement. Such attention to all these details is particularly relevant to palliative care units who have out-patient centres and day care facilities and regularly use voluntary transport.

Documentation

The need for accurate records and appropriate expenses claim forms for out-of-pocket expenses has been outlined above, but there are other documents which should form part of the support and management of all staff paid and unpaid. Great care must be taken in the way these documents are written and the terminology that is used.

The voluntary status of an individual can be jeopardized if certain words (illustrations are given below) are used that could persuade an employment tribunal (if a claim was made) that the standing of the person in the organization was that of an employee and not a volunteer.

Essential documents for the Voluntary Service Manager
A voluntary staff policy[2]

Just as it must have a policy document for its paid staff, every palliative care service should have a *voluntary staff policy document*. The purpose of this important document is to provide overall guidance and direction to staff and volunteers involved in the work of the service. The difference between the staff and volunteer's version will be in the words used. This is to ensure that volunteers have not entered into any contractual arrangement with the service which implies that they are employees rather than volunteers. The volunteer policy should be scrutinized by a lawyer to ensure that everything required is included and that the terminology is safe.

Other documents which should be part of the VSM's toolkit for safe and successful volunteer management include:

- An application form.[3]
- Induction form (see Appendix 2).
- Volunteer commitment or agreement form.[4]
- Volunteer assessment form.[5]
- Disciplinary and grievance procedures (usually included in the volunteer policy).
- An exit questionnaire.[6]

These documents all need to be carefully worded to ensure there is no confusion concerning paid and voluntary workers. They enable good support and supervision for volunteers and are a tool of control for the VSM. The wording in these documents need to be particularly accurate with no hint of words, such as *'contract,' 'employer', 'job description', 'grievance procedure'*, and *'dismissal'*, which could be wrongly construed as employment terms. Words which would be more applicable to a volunteer would be *'arrangement', 'organization', 'task list',*[7] *'arrangements if you have a complaint or are unhappy'*, and *'the ending of an arrangement'*. If courts or tribunals are involved with a difficult situation involving a volunteer they could construe that the terminology or method of payment is contractual and that the volunteer is an employee.[8]

Voluntary staff should not be doing the same tasks as paid staff. They should be carrying out duties which give added value to the service. As described elsewhere in this book, these might include running a coffee bar, maintaining the grounds, carrying out reception duties during out-of-office hours, assisting with fund-raising events, and many other supportive roles thus allowing the professional staff time and space to care for the patients and families which is at the core of palliative care.

It is bad practice for any service to bring in a volunteer to take the place of a paid member of staff who has left the organization. It is appreciated that many palliative care services could not continue without the services of many volunteers in both professional and support roles, but to replace paid staff by volunteers should not be considered. There are good legal reasons for this. Volunteers do not have to have the same commitment in terms of time given, do not have to give statutory times of notice of leaving the service, and do not have to follow the employment policies laid down. Filling a vacancy on the paid staff with a volunteer could lead to a lack of continuity of appropriate personnel carrying out the work of the unit.

Categories of volunteers

Depending on the structure of the palliative care service and whether it is independent or attached to a general hospital, there could be three main categories of volunteers:

1 Management Committee/Trustees.
2 Direct service volunteers (helping within the palliative care unit).
3 Charity shop volunteers and fund-raising volunteers.

Each of these three categories will be discussed in order and the duty of care, which is described in detail for direct service volunteers, should apply to *all* volunteers in each of the three categories.

Management Committee/Trustees

These volunteers are usually people of standing in the community and have professional qualifications relevant to the needs of the organization but do not carry out their duties under the management of the VSM. They are usually appointed to the Board of Management/Committees by the Board of Directors, their appointment being minuted at a Board Meeting, and in the case of Directors, ratified at the next Annual General Meeting of the 'company'. In the UK, if the palliative care service/hospice/organization is a company limited by guarantee, then each member of the Board of Directors must sign a form for Companies House. They are therefore accountable to that office. If the organization is unincorporated and is registered as a charity then the members of the Management Committee are accountable to the Inland Revenue (Scotland) or the Charities Commission (England and Wales). Directors who manage palliative care units attached to general hospitals will be accountable to the Health Trust or whichever organization manages the hospitals concerned. People who serve an organization in this way need to be aware of their legal responsibilities. The legal structure of most charities means that its members or Trustees can be responsible for meeting the liabilities of the charity. The organization should have a library of relevant legislation publications and should refer to them when issues of potential legal implications are being considered. Procedures should be in place to protect these individuals (see the section *Insurance policies*).

As members of a governing body they have many roles and responsibilities each with legal obligations:

♦ charity Trustees, if the organization is set up for charitable purposes;

♦ company directors, if it is registered as a company;

♦ employers, if the organization employs staff;

♦ owners and/or occupiers of premises;

♦ owners and/or users of vehicles;

♦ providers of services and/or goods;

♦ organizers of activities open to the public;

♦ publishers of publications, advertisements, and other materials.

Where should legal advice be sought?

A lawyer need not check *all* the documents used by the VSM but should be asked to check certain documents, such as the volunteer commitment/agreement, as well as the voluntary staff policy document and other complex matters. This will ensure that no contractual terms have been used and that the organization, by the introduction of such documentation is not contravening any equal opportunities policy or infringing any law such as the Human Rights Act.

This advice may be available from local lawyers/solicitors with experience in the voluntary sector, the local council for voluntary service or umbrella associations, such as the National Council for Voluntary Organisations (England and Wales) and the Scottish Council for Voluntary Organisations, which have an advice service.

Direct service volunteers

Volunteers who carry out regular duties in palliative care services should be covered by: (1) Health and Safety protection, and (2) insurance policies.

Health and safety protection

This is in place in most organizations, and should be applied to volunteers as well as employees. In UK, the Health and Safety at Work Act 1974 and its related legislation sets out what is required to protect employees of an organization. Areas in which volunteers are carrying out duties should be risk assessed and a document produced. Volunteers are then required to read this document and sign a form that they have done so (see Appendix 2). This should protect both the volunteers and the organization from litigation.

The basic requirements to comply with this Act are:

+ maintaining safe premises;
+ maintaining equipment properly, having proper safeguards for dangerous equipment, and ensuring that everyone who uses equipment is adequately and appropriately trained;
+ having a designated person trained in first aid;
+ having a health and safety policy (*in writing if there are more than four employees*);
+ ensuring the health and safety policy is read and signed by all employees and volunteers (*it is good practice to include volunteers although this is not legally required*);
+ carrying out an assessment of the risks posed by the premises, equipment or the work itself and developing a Health and Safety scheme to reduce the likelihood of risks happening or to reduce the effects if they do happen;
+ ensuring everyone knows their responsibilities in relation to Health and Safety, including their responsibility to carry out work carefully and not putting themselves or others at risk;
+ ensuring everyone knows their rights in relation to health and safety.

Further information is available from the local Health and Safety Executive office.

Insurance policies

Insurance for various reasons outlined below is essential and should be in place. They are likely to vary according to local conditions but the items discussed should have insurance cover. The volunteers in the course of their duties may be exposed to a variety of risks which may include:

1 Personal injury or death resulting from accidents and physical assault.
2 Claims against them for damage to property or personal injury for which they can be held legally liable.
3 Loss of or damage to personal property.

The reasons why insurance cover should be provided are obvious. Insurance is the main financial provision in the event of accidents to or by volunteers in the course of their duties. If the service fails to provide adequate protection, especially in increasingly litigious times, it may find itself in financial jeopardy as well as damaging its reputation.

Not only should VSMs be aware of what insurance is in place and the total amount of cover provided, but so should the volunteers themselves. In particular, they should also be informed if any restrictions to the insurance cover apply, such as participating in high-risk activities that are popular in some fund-raising events. It should be noted that having adequate and appropriate insurance cover does not absolve palliative care services, which have voluntary staff, from putting in place measures to minimize risk.

The palliative care service must have the following:

- *Vehicle insurance* for its own vehicles.
- *Buildings insurance* if it is a charity and owns its own buildings. If it rents or is buying a building the landlord or provider of the mortgage may also require this insurance.
- *Contents insurance* if it is a charity and has equipment or other contents of value.

Other insurance policies, which must be in place to protect individuals and the organization, are:

- **Employer's Liability**. This covers charity trustees and management committee members for death or injury to a volunteer or employee if specified within the policy. Volunteers who are helping the organization off-site can be covered by this insurance only if it is stated in the policy.

- **Trustee Indemnity**. This covers breach of professional duty, breach of trust and unintentional breach of confidentiality. It also covers negligent act, error or omission, misstatement, misleading statement, breach of warranty of authority, slander, and defamation. This type of policy only covers acts made in good faith by any directors, officers, trustees or committee members, employees or volunteers.

- **Public and Products Liability**. This will cover volunteers against claims by a third party for death or injury or damage to property belonging to them. It provides cover for products sold by the charity (e.g. in cafes and restaurants), as well as second-hand goods sold in charity shops. This insurance also covers the public who have access to the premises, such as visitors of patients and anyone attending any other activity like coffee mornings or open days, and education courses and clients of the shops and cafes. Agencies which fund palliative care establishments, especially Local Authorities, often require this to be in place.

- **Personal Accident**. This provides fixed benefits in the event of an accident while on the business of the charity. Cover is usually given up to the age of 85. This insurance for volunteers provides compensation over and above what there is a legal liability to do; thus giving volunteers extra protection against accident. This means that although already protected by public liability insurance the volunteer is also given extra cover with this personal accident insurance. *This is an important insurance to consider providing as it does provide special care for the voluntary staff.*

♦ **Motor Vehicle Insurance**. The palliative care service should ensure that there is appropriate insurance cover for volunteers who drive motor vehicles, whether hired or owned by it. Volunteers who drive their own cars as part of their duty in the organization should inform their insurance company in writing. They should also state that they will not be in receipt of any profit for their voluntary work, only having expenses remunerated at or below the mileage rate set by the Taxation Department if applicable. The '*no-claims bonus*' of a volunteer who may be involved in an accident while driving on behalf of the organization should also be protected by insurance. Many insurance companies have the 'no claims bonus' as a standard part of the cover, but the palliative care service must enable this to be in place for those volunteer drivers who do not carry such insurance.

It is essential that *all* volunteer drivers inform their insurance company that they are driving for the hospice or palliative care unit. In most cases, driving of patients is considered 'social' driving and there is no penalty, but in the author's experience it has been known for a higher premium to been levied to accommodate this 'extra' driving of patients on a weekly basis. It should be emphasized that this is a rare occurrence.

♦ **Professional Indemnity Insurance**. This covers the organization in respect of legal liabilities for injury, damage or financial loss resulting from giving incorrect advice or information. These liabilities may also apply even if the advice is given free of charge (e.g. when volunteers are involved with telephone helplines). Liability can arise in respect of both written and oral advice.

It is very important that the insurance policies taken out by the organization should be carefully worded to ensure that volunteers are always covered as well as are employees, Trustees, and the public. Specialist insurers are available who can give advice to organizations in the voluntary sector.

Charity shop and fund-raising volunteers

We discussed volunteers serving as Trustees or on committees. We now turn to volunteers working in charity shop or as fund-raising volunteers. Most of their duties for the palliative care service are performed outside the main premises but nevertheless they should be cared for as outlined above under *Direct service volunteers*. In particular, they must be adequately insured (see above) as they go about their duties, and the Health and Safety issues reassessed for the environment which they are in. This may be the responsibility of the VSM or management or the organizer of the event. In most cases, Public Liability Insurance or the organization would cover the volunteer, but in this case it must be written into the policy. However, depending on the event special insurance may be required. Local legal and insurance advice should be sought when volunteers are helping in venues outside the normal premises of the palliative care service.

Volunteers who help the organization by working in their own homes need to contact their home insurers to advise them of the details of their policy. All property in the house that belongs to the palliative care service, such as computer equipment, printers, fax machine, etc., should be insured by the service.

Legislation

Equal opportunities policy

Although not universally legally binding, such a policy should be in place. The statement could read:

> (*Name of organization*) operates a policy that no person or employee receives less favourable treatment on the grounds of sex, disability, marital status, age, race (including colour, nationality, ethnic or national origin), creed, sexuality, responsibility for dependants, political party or trade union membership or activity, HIV/AIDS status or is disadvantaged by conditions or requirements which cannot be shown or justifiable.

Human Rights Act (UK)

This Act stems from the European Convention of Human Rights which is a product of the Council of Europe. The Act enables UK citizens and residents to enforce the European Convention of Human Rights in domestic courts.

Convention rights include the:

+ right to respect for private and family life, home, and correspondence;
+ right to freedom of thought, conscience, and religion;
+ right to freedom of expression;
+ right not to be discriminated against in the exercise of another Convention article.

This Act applies directly to public authorities and private bodies including charities and other voluntary organizations which carry out a public function. It is likely that palliative care units and independent hospices by caring for their patients are fulfilling a public function and as such it is essential those functions comply with the Convention rights.

Rehabilitation of Offenders Act

This Act has an exemption clause which allows some convictions to become spent after a certain time. [The Rehabilitation of Offenders Act 1974 (exceptions) Order 1975 (SI 1975 No. 1023).] This clause *does not* apply in health care organizations such as palliative care units. An application form for volunteers in palliative care should have a statement that invites the prospective volunteer to reveal any past convictions spent or unspent. This exemption clause also does not apply when volunteers may be involved with children under 18 years of age. It would be good practice to make it clear that disclosure of a conviction would not necessarily disqualify a person from working as a volunteer but only in a health care environment or with young children.

Police Act 1997 (part V of the UK Police Act 1997)

This allows access to police records and applies to employees and volunteers. This Act is particularly relevant where children or vulnerable adults are the client group and an enhanced criminal record certificate is available in this case. The UK government is likely to make it unlawful to employ a person with certain criminal convictions for any work closely involved with children. Police checks would be an important part of the recruitment procedures for children's hospices (see Chapter 10). In the UK it is not binding at this time for charities and other voluntary organizations to make police checks on employees or volunteers except for individuals serving in a regulated position. This would include, for example, trusteeship of children's charities. Regulated positions are defined in the Criminal Justice and Court Services Act 2000 s36.

Foreign nationals as volunteers

There can be restrictions depending on local conditions for people applying for voluntary work abroad. Within the EU/EEA people can move around undertaking paid or unpaid work. In other parts of the world it may be that special arrangements can be made to allow foreign nationals to apply for voluntary work.

Asylum and Immigration Act 1995

In the UK, this Act makes it an offence for an employer to employ a person who is not entitled to work in the UK. This Act does not apply to people who are genuine (unpaid) volunteers as distinct from paid employees. In some countries, however, people who are applying for refugee status are not entitled to take on any paid *or* unpaid work. This restriction can be overcome depending on how long the application for asylum has been pending and can be waived after suitable application to the appropriate government department. The question of expenses for asylum seekers when volunteering must be carefully controlled so that they are not perceived as employees. They should only be granted genuine reimbursement supported by receipts and must not receive any other benefits other than the training required to carry out their duty.

The rules that apply to asylum seekers, will vary from country to country across the world and are changing regularly, but care must be taken and advice sought before they are introduced as volunteers into an organization. This Act is presently (2002) under review in the UK. Further information is available in the UK from the National Council for Volunteering (0800–028–8304).

Data Protection Acts

When a new volunteer joins an organization, personal details need to be taken and placed on file on a computer database and hard copy is usually also placed on file. The volunteer should give permission for their details to be stored in this way. This can be accomplished by having a statement regarding this on the volunteer's application form which they must sign. The volunteer should have access at any time to this information and be assured that all details will be kept in confidence. In the UK, there is a Data Protection Act 1998 that applies to employers and employees. Once again, although voluntary workers are not discussed in the Act, best practice procedures should be adopted to encompass the rights of volunteers to have their personal file kept secure.

Much of the legislation referred to above is based on UK Law although some comes from European Law. It should be emphasized that two crucial aspects of the above information are that:

1 Adequate, all-encompassing insurance is available for all concerned in the organization whether working and helping within the buildings or out in the community. If there is any doubt then specialist advice should be taken from the local voluntary organization service.

2 Legal advice should be sought on important documents such as the voluntary staff policy and volunteer agreements. There could be other occasions when legal advice is necessary. The Voluntary Service Manager should not hesitate to seek legal help if in doubt about the implementation of any new policy. The consequences of not doing so could be very serious indeed.

Conclusion

It is hoped that the reader will find interest and guidance on best practice procedures on the headings discussed. Although volunteers are rarely mentioned in the substance of many laws defined for the workplace, it is clearly best practice to care for volunteers as if they were paid employees as the organization has responsibility for their welfare and security. It will be necessary therefore wherever palliative care is practised that awareness and investigation of local employment law is seriously considered.

Palliative care units worldwide each depend on hundreds of volunteers to support their staff, to enhance the environment, and help with funding. It is in their interests to keep the volunteers happy in their duties and safe in their premises.

The contents of this chapter are believed to be accurate at the time of going to press. It must be made emphasized that legal requirements change and evolve year on year and that each organization must take responsibility to discover what the rights of their employees and volunteers are. It would be prudent to have legal advice at all stages when implementing new procedures and structures within an organization. This is especially true when producing documentation for staff and volunteers as part of their management.

Acknowledgements

My thanks to Sandy Adirondack for access to her information on legal matters affecting voluntary organizations, which has been adapted for this chapter, and to the Edinburgh Volunteer Exchange for helpful advice.

Appendix 1
Specimen Health and Safety Policy document

A Health and Safety Policy document should contain the following headings:

1. The policy statement of intent for the organization which should be signed by a director or senior manager with responsibility for health and safety

2. Health and Safety responsibilities which explains who has responsibility for what. Items from the Health and Safety at Work Act 1974 are usually quoted and Regulation 12 of the Management of Health and Safety at Work Regulations 1992 also quoted.

3. A list of instructions to paid and unpaid staff is required. For example, 'All our employees and voluntary staff must: (a) comply with the Health and Safety Policy, (b) avoid any improvisations of any form which could create an unnecessary risk to their personal safety and to the safety of others'.

4. Safety Rules should be listed. There should be subheadings such as:

   - Working practices.
   - Warning signs and other notices.
   - Working conditions/environment.
   - Fire precautions with fire procedure explained.
   - Employer's transport.
   - Accident/illnesses.
   - Health.
   - Hygiene.
   - Protective clothing and equipment.
   - Drugs and medicine.
   - Food hygiene, preparation, and storage.

5. What to do in the case of an accident at work. This should contain:

   - Details of the accident.
   - Who was injured.
   - Kind of injury.
   - Action required.

This document should be laid out clearly and simple to read. A form should accompany it and should be signed and dated by every new employee or volunteer after they have read and understood the document. An example of this form is shown in Appendix 2.

Appendix 2

1. Sample of form for the Health and Safety policy

PRIVATE AND CONFIDENTIAL

(*Name of organization*)

Please read the notes below and sign this form.

We have now formulated our Health and Safety at Work Policy and Procedures as legally required and this is to inform you that those sections of the Policy which affect our volunteers are contained in the Volunteer Services Health and Safety document which is usually kept in the:

VOLUNTEER OFFICE

Clearly, we will do all in our power to ensure the health, safety and welfare of our employees and volunteers and we look to them to abide by the health and safety standards laid down.

You should now read the Volunteer Services Health and Safety Handbook which is part of your Volunteer Commitment. Please discuss any queries you may have with the Volunteer Services Manager.

I have read the Volunteer Services Health and Safety Handbook and understand and accept its contents as forming part of my Volunteer Commitment. I will keep myself informed of its contents.

Volunteer's signature:_____   Date:_____

Please return this form to the Volunteer Service Manager

2. Sample of form for induction of volunteers

VOLUNTEER OFFICE
INDUCTION OF NEW VOLUNTEERS TO THE HOSPICE

Notes for Volunteer Service Manager and Team Co-ordinators

When a new volunteer joins a team, please ensure that they: **Info. given**

(a) Know about signing in and signing out at reception   ☐

(b) Have been given, and are wearing their name badge   ☐

(c) Know location of cloakroom, security lockers, and toilets   ☐

(d) Have read and understood the fire drill notice at their work
station, and know where alarms/extinguishers are located   ☐

(e) Have read the Employee Handbook and signed the
Health and Safety form   ☐

(f) Know where and to whom to report an accident   ☐

(g) What to do if they are unable to attend (e.g. holiday/illness)   ☐

(h) Remember to inform the Volunteer Office of any changes
in circumstances (e.g. name/address/telephone numbers)   ☐

(i) Have a copy of the guidelines appropriate for their
particular task   ☐

(j) Know at any time, if they need to air any anxieties,
problems or grievances to contact the Volunteer Office   ☐

Volunteer signature:_____

Volunteer Services Manager/
Team Co-ordinator signature:_____

Date:_____

References

1. McCurley S and Lynch R (1998). Appendix B. In *Essential volunteer management* (2nd edn), p. 211. Directory of Social Change, London.
2. Ibid., pp. 187–99.
3. Ibid., p. 205.
4. Ibid., p. 208.
5. Ibid., p. 214.
6. Ibid., p. 216.
7. Ibid., p. 204.
8. Ibid., p. 506.

Recommended reading

Adirondack S and Sinclair Taylor J (2001). *The voluntary sector legal handbook* (2nd edn). Directory of Social Change, London.

McCurley S and Lynch R (1998). *Essential volunteer management* (2nd edn). Directory of Social Change, London

Useful organizations

Scottish Council for Voluntary Organisations, 18/19 Claremont Crescent, Edinburgh EH7 4DQ, UK.

National Council for Voluntary Organisations, Regent's Wharf, 8 All Saint's Street, London N1 9RL, UK.

Volunteer Development Scotland, 72 Murray Place Stirling, FK8 2BX, UK.

'Involve' Managing Volunteers In Palliative Care, c/o Help the Hospices, 34–44 Britannia Street, London WC1X 9JG, UK.

Help the Hospices, 34–44 Britannia Street, London WC1X 9JG, UK.

Chapter 14

Ethical issues for the Volunteer Service Manager

It cannot be denied that ethics is a huge topic. It is a topic that has been explored from many perspectives such as religious, business, medical, social, environmental, scientific, and philosophical. Each highlights new theories and guidelines. This chapter does not aim to examine all ethical issues in detail but rather to focus on key areas as they relate to volunteers within a palliative care service. It will outline issues and raise discussion points for Voluntary Service Managers and their volunteers to explore further and develop in relation to their specific context. It will pose questions that might usefully be explored in joint training sessions with volunteers and staff.

What do people mean when they talk about ethics and ethical issues? This chapter defines ethics as 'the moral principles or standards of people's conduct'. The moral standards that make up an individual's ethics are absorbed from a number of different areas: religion, nature, individuality, and society.[1] Values can be said to be both objective and subjective. Acceptance of certain behaviours differs between individuals. What one person finds acceptable someone else may find offensive. Another problem relates to how individuals interpret ethical activity. This will depend on the influencing factors that have affected the individuals involved in any particular situation.

Some ethical standards may be stronger than others. For example, it is generally accepted that it is wrong to kill. However, even the strongest of values can be debated at different levels. What about self-defence? What about abortion? What about so-called mercy killings? Is there ever a situation when it is acceptable to kill? Standards vary not only between communities and countries, but also between individuals.

This chapter acknowledges that each palliative care unit may have a different approach to ethical standards. It does not offer right or wrongs but offers questions for each unit to explore. The important message is that the ethical expectations of the volunteer team should complement and mirror that of the health professionals' codes of conduct. In order to achieve this goal guidance and training will certainly be required.

This chapter reviews the issues surrounding ethical guidance, it explores key areas of ethical concerns which should be addressed by a unit in regard to volunteers, highlights the structures required to support ethical guidance, and finally suggests some methods of relaying and explaining the ethic standards to a volunteer team.

Ethical issues in people management

Volunteer management is a specialized area of people management—hence this book. Volunteers generate substantial ethical considerations, which are founded within the debate of: 'How much and what can we actually ask someone to do if we aren't paying them?' These issues have been raised throughout the book but it is good practice to review the issues not only from an operational or strategic perspective but also an ethical one.

A hospice or palliative care unit and its Trustees have to ask some core questions, for example:

1. Why should it use volunteers?
2. What structure, planning and resources need to be committed to effective volunteer services management?
3. What tasks can/should volunteers undertake?
4. What value is placed on the work of volunteers?
5. Management of volunteers.

Volunteer involvement

Why can charities get away with free labour? What has created the expectation that charities *must* involve volunteers? Do they do so to benefit the patient, the volunteer, the unit or is it a multiway process? Do volunteers enhance and supplement services or do they replace paid staff during a financial crisis? What makes a position paid—how is this decision arrived at? These important questions are addressed in several chapters of this book

A charity (the Trustees, Board of Directors, and Management) should brainstorm and review what benefits they receive by involving volunteers and then ask if the unit is satisfied that these benefits/decisions are ethical? The organization should be able to list specific benefits on which to base ethical statements explaining why the unit involves volunteers. These statements can then direct future volunteer management decisions.

Volunteer service provision

Once the decision has been made to include volunteers the organization has to show commitment to supporting the decision and providing adequate resources to ensure the volunteer services can operate effectively. Volunteer services are not free. How ethically acceptable is it to accept individuals to perform certain roles without the resources to complete the tasks? Are volunteers seen as part of the team or are they 'just' volunteers? Are volunteers expected/permitted to get it wrong or are they expected to meet the unit's standards? Volunteers represent the unit—has the unit explored its ethical standards?

The message that management gives regarding the value of volunteer contributions will influence staff, in addition to the personal experience of volunteers. Do staff feel threatened by volunteers? Establishing ethical statements of volunteer involvement will cover these issues but recurrent problems can be expected and must be addressed.

Volunteer tasks

Many issues integrate with each other. The type of tasks offered to volunteers might raise status but may lead to increased staff insecurity. Are volunteers only good enough to pour tea and go round with a trolley (not wishing to demean those tasks in any way)? Or can the model be expanded to utilize the skills and experience of individual volunteers or the ability to train a group of volunteers? Some hospices and palliative care units are currently debating whether volunteers should help with hands-on patient care (see Chapter 8 describing this in South Africa). Some units have recruited trained nurses as volunteers—if this is done, should the organization use the volunteers as part of the nursing establishment or as additional resources? (see Chapter 12). To whom should they be accountable—the Nursing Director or the Voluntary Service Manager? In one Budapest hospital unit they state that wards would have closed if they did not have the practical help of volunteers. Is there anything wrong with this approach in your environment? It may not be suitable for all units. Is there a right or wrong? If volunteers are involved in a professional capacity are they up to date with current practices and how is this measured? Will the unit pay for further training or professional updating? Are the volunteers expected to keep themselves up to date? Have the volunteers got professional indemnity insurance? Who pays for it?

Role boundaries

For some volunteers, boundaries will prove a difficult concept to comprehend. It can be hard to see the wider picture of an organization if the volunteer only comes into the unit for a few hours each week. The Volunteer Service Manager needs to ensure each volunteer understands where their role begins and ends and how that role fits into the wider picture of the work done in the palliative care unit by both the volunteers and the professional staff. The issue of boundaries is such an important one that a VSM will need to spend a lot of time explaining and re-emphasizing it.

Most palliative care units break down volunteer roles into defined areas of involvement which enable volunteers to be trained for specific areas of care (e.g. bereavement care, community visiting, etc.). The VSM should provide clear guidelines for the volunteers which give details of:

◆ The tasks required in the role.
◆ Training required for the role.
◆ The care team the role is associated with.
◆ The type of patients the role is involved with (e.g. in-patients, day care, etc.).

- The recommended role shifts.
- The role supervisor/volunteer team leader to whom the volunteer can refer issues.
- Where the remit of the role begins and finishes, where referrals to other team members can be made by the supervisor/team leader.
- The standards required of the role.

It is critically important that volunteers do not cross boundaries with other team members. If a volunteer performs tasks that do not fall within the role remit, they are potentially putting the patient at risk, and possibly usurping the role of fellow volunteers. They may inadvertently place other volunteers under pressure to follow suit if the patient requests the same from other volunteers. Examples include drivers taking patients home, stopping off at the shops, or taking the patients for excursions rather than going straight home. The volunteer must accept the level of professionalism required for the role. Volunteers represent the charity and they must adhere to the standards that the organization works to. One member of the team, whether paid or unpaid cannot offer a patient all the assistance they require. The volunteer must recognize and acknowledge how their role fits into the bigger picture. Much as they might be tempted to offer help outwith their volunteer remit they must accept that others will be expected to do that as part of the comprehensive care people receive in a hospice or palliative care unit.

Volunteer management

Some charities can be so desperate for help that they will accept anyone who volunteers. A clinical unit has an ethical responsibility to its patients that all staff and volunteers are selected carefully and trained to effectively perform the tasks requested of them in a professional manner (see Chapters 4 and 5). The screening process should include an ethical examination. Should a volunteer be rejected on the grounds of ethical incompatibility? The VSM has a responsibility to ensure the volunteer team is given training, guidance and support on ethical issues (see Chapter 5).

If a volunteer opposes or is unhappy with the unit's ethical or operational practices should the hospice or palliative care unit discipline or dismiss volunteers? Unlike other team members they are usually not covered by a professional code of conduct, but they are expected in many cases to follow policy and procedure. Volunteers are committed to the cause but they are not contracted with the unit. What happens when a volunteer's view of appropriate care differs from that of the organization? Is it possible or desirable or practicable to sack a volunteer? Sometimes, the question might be: 'Is the patient safe if the volunteer stays?'

When standards of any description are established a reward or punishment system often follows. Volunteers may be rewarded for adhering to ethical standards to encourage future behaviour. Reward may be verbal recognition or include development opportunities.

Punishment for non-adherence to ethical and other standards must be clearly stated at the *beginning* of the selection/training process so that individuals understand the consequences of any action. Punishment should be fair and aimed to protect patients from such individual's actions, to deter similar breaches of agreements, to assist the individual to improve their ability to adhere to standards, and to deter others following any examples.

Action that might be taken when a volunteer breaks the ethical code or otherwise does not meet the standards set, might involve reassigning a volunteer to another team or another role until the organization is confident that no further breaches will occur. It might involve shadowing other trustworthy volunteers as part of a revision training scheme. If the volunteer's behaviour does not alter, the organization will need to consider which criteria are required in order to ask a volunteer to leave the organization. Palliative care is a specialized field; it is not suitable for everyone. It should not be assumed just because volunteers are prepared to involve themselves in such an environment that they are suitable candidates. Sometimes, it is not until volunteers have experienced a volunteer role that the complete picture of their suitability or unsuitability emerges.

Clinical ethical issues

Volunteers within a hospice or palliative care units are involved with particularly vulnerable patients and their relatives, and may have access to delicate personal information. Palliative care focuses upon the quality of life, achieved through patient-centred care provided by all the members of a team, which includes the volunteers. Ethical issues are an integral component of caring services and volunteers should be informed by the unit of the ethical expectations required of them.

What are these clinical ethical issues? The National Association of Social Workers' broad ethical principles are based on six core Social Work values of service: social justice, dignity, worth of the person, importance of human relationships, integrity, and competence. These principles are broken down into a further forty-six ethical standards.[2] The scope is endless, especially within a complex area such as palliative care. Here, we shall look at just a few basic ethical issues whilst offering suggestions and challenges for further discussion at unit level.

Confidentiality

Confidentiality within a health setting may be a new concept to some volunteers. It is much more than someone divulging a piece of information without permission to do so. It is important that the organization, through the VSM, explicitly explains what it means by confidentiality. It should state what the unit expects of the volunteers in this matter, what information volunteers in different roles may have access to, whether or not they may attend clinical meetings where patients are discussed. It might further be asked if volunteers should ever have access to case records? What mechanisms are in place for the volunteer to pass their observations on to the member of staff in charge of the patient's care? Are the volunteers certain of which information must be passed on to the team? Are volunteers aware of the boundaries of confidentiality?

For example, volunteers might be asked to gather information from patients but the volunteer, like the VSM, should be made aware of the importance of the patient's right to privacy. Volunteers should never enquire about private matters that are not relevant to the patient's care and that the patient does not wish to discuss. There should be clear guidelines regarding the disclosure of private information. Some charities state that all information given by patients must be passed on and that the VSM or volunteer team leader will take the relevant issues forward. Others, such as volunteer chaplains, may require general information without the detail.

What matters is that each unit must decided on an appropriate policy, which may differ between volunteer roles, but takes into account ethical and legal considerations. The policy should also state any exceptions to the rule, for example, if the information places the patient or another party at risk, or it may include medical information. It is the responsibility of the hospice/palliative care unit to ensure that it provides support to allow the volunteer to manage the level of confidentiality within which they operate. No member of the team, whether paid or unpaid should carry too many burdens on their shoulders.

Patients, too, sometimes need to be made aware of the issues surrounding the disclosure of confidential information. Volunteers need to be shown how to handle this delicate issue. For example, when patients ask volunteers if they can tell them something confidential volunteers should be recommended to give a courteous but guarded reply such as '…by all means, I would be willing to listen but depending on what you tell me I may need to pass any information back to the hospice team if it will affect your care'. The patient can then decide on the action that he/she wishes to take. It is important that the respect and the good of the patient are at the heart of any communication.

Other confidentiality issues include discussing confidential matters in private surroundings away from the hospice; care when conveying information via telephone, fax, or e-mail; discrete disposal of confidential records, reports, and letters; protection of confidentiality of deceased patients; total confidentiality of all personal information outside of the health care setting; confidential issues relating to any policy changes or developments in the hospice and details about donors and mailing lists. At times, there can be a fine line between a volunteer having a healthy interest and being nosy!

The VSM has a responsibility to make sure the guidelines are formulated and communicated, along with the consequences of breach of confidentiality

Relationship boundaries

Relationships are rarely straightforward. In a vulnerable, emotive environment the unit must have in place clear guidelines to promote professional—quality volunteer relations with patient/client, professional staff, and the unit.

Some everyday scenarios and questions arising from them are listed below to illustrate this need for guidelines and to promote discussion in volunteer teams.

♦ Should volunteers be allowed to see patients outside the unit? Usually not, but does this apply to all units? What are the issues here?

♦ Should volunteers form personal relationships with patients beyond the normal friendly relationship that exists in the hospice itself? What are the issues here as they affect the patient and as they affect the volunteer service? What should the unit do in such a situation?

♦ Do the volunteers understand the dangers of becoming too friendly with patients—from a personal, patient, carer, family perspective? What is 'too friendly'?

♦ Does the unit encourage or permit personal touching? What are the issues here?

♦ How should a unit and its management respond if a volunteer is named as a beneficiary in a patient's will?

♦ Do volunteers need to attend a patient's funeral? Should they be encouraged to do so?

♦ If volunteers are offered gifts by patients or their families should they ever accept them? If so, need they always declare them and if the are not permitted to accept them, how should they deal with the offer? Nursing teams are often given boxes of chocolates—should volunteers be treated differently?

♦ When are 'friendly' and well-meaning gestures by volunteers not helpful or appropriate? How is it possible for a volunteer to become too deeply involved? Examples might be the volunteer driver who offers to take the patient's laundry home to do it for them or the one who bakes a cake for the patient. Another might be the well-meaning volunteer who offers her husband's skills as a solicitor to help the patient with some legal problem. What of the volunteer who offers to do the shopping for a patient or who expects a friendly kiss each time a patient visits the day hospice? What are the hazards of such gestures?

♦ How can a volunteer be effective in his/her role without becoming involved at a personal emotional level? What personal protection techniques can the unit teach its volunteer team?

Relationships between volunteers and members of the professional (paid) staff are important for all concerned. Whose 'side' is the volunteer on—the patient's or the unit's? The volunteer may be tempted to adopt a patient advocacy role in preference to a loyalty one towards the unit, its staff, and its policies. Ethically, the volunteer should usually represent the unit and support the unit's policies as well as its strengths and limitations.

As in all professional relationships, volunteers should not demean, belittle or implicitly criticize other volunteers or staff members when speaking to patients, relatives or other members of the hospice team. It is the responsibility of the VSM to explain this, giving examples of how easily, and usually unintentionally, it can happen. What is ethically necessary is for mutual respect, appreciation of the skills and work of others, and speaking of others as we would like people to speak of us. In a word—respect.

Patient freedom

In many countries, the culture is now such that individuals and the society they form are free to make personal decisions and act accordingly, within legal, social, and environmental constraints—'autonomy'. Do we find patient autonomy within a palliative care unit? Has the unit or individual members of its staff or informal carers 'taken over' patients' freedom? Can action performed 'in the best interest of the patient' actually restrict patient choice? This is a real ethical question that must asked. Is there a danger that a hospice/palliative care unit can become paternalistic?

Volunteers should be helped to understand the difference between being an advocate for a patient and being a spokesperson. Volunteers cannot assume they know or understand a patient's needs or take control away from the patient. Some patients are prepared to accept situations that others find intolerable. Others want to continue to make decisions affecting their lives while others happily delegate that responsibility to someone else. Volunteers may need to be helped to accept the wishes of the patient and let the patient control the situation, however ill-advised that may appear to the volunteer.

Volunteers should be given the opportunity to discuss issues of how well-meant actions can de-power patients, to review the notion of patient autonomy, and the consequences of patient choice regarding treatment or care plans. Useful examples might be the patient who refuses to go into a nursing home, the effects of overpowering carers on a patient, how limited resources may effect patient choice, the occasions when a patient's freedom of choice should be overridden, the effects of patient choice on others, those situations where health professionals put patients' wishes before their wellbeing and vica versa, and the limits this may impose on what the care team can do for the patient. Understanding the principle of respect for an individual will help focus a volunteer's response to patients.

Equality of care

Can care be truly equitable given resource limitations? It is important that volunteers treat all patients as equals within the confinements of resources. Volunteers, like all members of the professional care team, should not differentiate between patients/carers on the grounds of ethnicity, religion, sexual orientation, diagnosis, education, etc. Obvious as this may seem volunteers may find themselves more attracted to caring for people of the same social class as themselves or from the same educational or cultural background. They may share some interests. Conversation can be easier. Conversely, as many have discovered, it is easy to discriminate on grounds of colour or religion or because of the nature of their illness or sexual orientation and any societal stigma attached to it. Volunteers should make every endeavour not to be prejudiced but to accept people for who they are. They must try to detach personal preconceptions or feelings. If a volunteer finds a situation too difficult it may be appropriate for the VSM to reassign the volunteer temporarily, without attaching any blame on them.

Honesty

We are taught to tell the truth. It is soon evident that some situations would be made easier with a small lie or two. Telling the truth can be complicated, and often more difficult than telling untruths, but honesty is a fundamental feature of palliative care and as relevant to volunteers as other professionals.

Volunteers must be informed of policies on informing patients of diagnosis, prognosis, care plans, etc. Volunteers should also be made aware of their role in the communication process. As stressed already, volunteers must know to whom to pass on a query, how much information they need to perform a task, and topics they may discuss with patients. This will protect volunteers in many difficult situations. It is the unit's responsibility to nurture an open, no-blame environment which will encourage volunteers and staff to admit to mistakes, to be as honest with each other as with their patients. The issue can be complex and touches on such issues as duty of care, respect for an individual, and patient empowerment.

Imposing views

Although guidelines and care practices cannot work in isolation volunteers should be helped to understand the dangers of operating according to their own ethical stance or promoting/imposing their own personal beliefs and values.

A common function of a volunteer role is to sit and chat with patients. During the course of a conversation a number of issues may arise. It is important that volunteers do not purposefully raise controversial issues or steer the conversation where the patient does not want it to go. The volunteer must not impose their views on to a patient, whether it be about religion, politics, sexual orientation, or anything else. The volunteer's role is to listen—no easy task but immensely important in palliative care

What is 'reasonable conduct' for a volunteer? The level of behaviour the unit should expect from its volunteers will vary depending on the culture in which the unit operates but the expectations and behaviour of the volunteer team should reflect that of the professional team. Striking the balance between legalistic rules and regulations and potential unruly individualistic morality is difficult but open discussions of conflict and development will promote ownership of practices throughout the team.

Additional bio-ethical considerations

Bio-ethics—'life ethics'—relate to the association between a patient and the medical/clinical professions. Palliative care is engulfed with clinical ethical issues, few of them unique to palliative care but many of them highlighted because of the nature of palliative care and its patients. Volunteers within such a setting may themselves never be involved with them but should certainly should be aware of them and be reassured that they are addressed by the Trustees, management, and the professional care team. Just as the latter addresses them so might some of the points in the box usefully be discussed on training course for volunteers.

Topics for discussion in training session

♦ The potential conflict between the responsibility to promote health, prevent illness, restore health, and alleviate suffering. What do these mean in the context of a hospice/palliative care service?
♦ Resuscitation policy. Is there ever a place for resuscitation in a palliative care unit?
♦ Sedation practices. Is sedation a form of euthanasia?
♦ Accepting a patient's decision not to accept treatment or care.
♦ Conflicts between patient's and family's wishes.
♦ Discussing diagnosis and prognosis.
♦ Level of information given to patients and carers. Who decides?
♦ Consent issues. Is there such a thing as 'informed consent'?
♦ Dealing with a patient's denial of the nature of their illness.
♦ Organ donation.
♦ Legal requirements regarding care.
♦ Research, drug trials, current medical treatment, and human experimentation.
♦ Euthanasia, assisted suicide, mercy killings, and allowing people to die.
♦ Allocation of medical resources.

Business ethics

Business ethics involves the creation and maintenance of good working relationships between employees, volunteers, business, and service users. Palliative care units operate within a business as well as a health setting.

Although not legally 'contracted employees', volunteers have the right to fairness, honesty, truth telling, security, and consultation. In return, volunteers are required to be honest and truthful, to behave fair and justly, to be sincere, and not to discriminate, to be trustworthy, to admit to errors, to fulfil tasks to their full ability, and to be loyal and committed to the hospice or palliative care unit.

The unit has an ethical responsibility to define and explain what it expects of volunteers and what its responsibility is to its volunteers, in exactly the same way as it must do for its paid staff.

'Whistleblowing' is not a user-friendly term but refers to individuals informing the relevant authority of malpractice. Issues could relate to colleagues' mistakes, poor standards of care, breech of policy, etc. It must be asked if it is ethical for team members to 'tell tales' on colleagues? Is whistleblowing protecting patients or the unit or both? Once again, volunteers should be aware of the channels of communication and the possibility of approaching top management if they have an issue that they believe should be dealt with at that level. Whatever process is put in place for communicating malpractice, it should be confidential, discrete, and offer protection to the informant.

Policies, procedures, and ethical issues

The VSM should provide opportunities to discuss with both his/her colleagues and volunteers ethical considerations in line with unit practices. Most units will have policies on most of the issues in this chapter. The policies should act as a guide for the volunteers. In a situation where personal ethical standards conflict with unit practice the volunteer must be informed that, when working for the unit, unit practice overrides *personal* ethical standards.

Whatever systems are put in place to govern volunteers' behaviour should they be as formal as for paid staff? When should units raise ethical issues with volunteers? Many units do so at induction, and thereafter rely on goodwill and personal character. Is this relaxed, informal approach good enough? Each unit must decide for itself.

Some hospices and palliative care units outline confidentiality guidelines that are signed by a volunteer, provide an induction booklet or training detailing boundary issues, and guidance on topics, such as gifts, etc. There are many ways of approaching the subject.

The existence of these policies, guidelines, and legislation will help but will not make an ethical problem go away, especially if patients are unclear to the type of acceptable demands to be made of a volunteer. The VSM needs to coach and support the volunteer team through individual ethical dilemmas and report back to the management and even Trustees regarding potential practice development or alteration.

Codes of conduct

Industries set standards of behaviour often referred to as 'codes of conduct'. The health sector is no different: examples include the UK Central Council code of professional conduct for nursing, midwifery and health visiting or the National Association of Social Workers code of ethics.

Ethics is a common subject on many health and social care courses. Most nurses, doctors, chaplains, social workers, etc. are required to sign a code of ethics before they are registered to practise their profession. Maintaining appropriate standards of moral conduct is everyone's responsibility. As mentioned previously, each person's interpretation of moral conduct may differ. A code of conduct generates unity of activity within a group.

The question could be asked whether volunteers should sign a code of conduct? One approach could be to establish an ethical statement/code of conduct for the entire hospice or palliative care unit—a code of conduct that reflects the essence of the professional codes but which unifies the unit's approach and applies to all team members, whether clinical, administrative, paid or unpaid. In an environment where a variety of different professionals and non-professionals work together, a specific organizational statement could ensure that patient care is provided consistently and the good name of the establishment is maintained. This statement can then be communicated to the whole team, whether paid or unpaid, as well as to patients and other service users

When establishing an ethical statement the charity must consider the consequences of such statements and the decisions, acts, and rules that are established. The statements should be established with the best interest of all involved parties, for example, employees, volunteers, patients, and families, etc.

The key features of any code of conduct should include.

- that it is rational but not devoid of emotion;
- that it is logical, but not rigid and inflexible;
- that it applies to all humanity but especially applicable to practical situations;
- that it is capable of being taught and being communicated;
- that it facilitates resolving conflicts amongst people, and defining duties and obligations.[3]

References

1. Thiroux J (1998). Ethics theory and practice (6th edn). Prentice Hall, London.
2. National Association of Social Workers (2001)., *Code of ethics*. http//www.nasawdc.org/code/ethics.htm
3. Thiroux J (1998), p. 177.

Glossary of terms

Alternative therapies   These, as the term implies, are therapies that are promoted as, and claimed to be, alternatives to traditional medicine. Because, as yet, no evidence has been presented to show that they are effective as claimed, and because in some cases harm has been shown to result from their use, they are not approved of, or prescribed by doctors.

Chief Executive   This is the recognized term for the most senior member of staff, responsible and reporting to the Board of Directors/Governors/Trustees whose task is to oversee the implementation of the decisions and policies of that body. The title is sometimes lengthened to Chief Executive Officer

Community palliative care service   Several reasons lie behind the decision to change the traditional term 'home care service' to 'community palliative care service'. It recognizes that people under care in the community may be in their own homes or those of relatives or in nursing homes. Now that there are so many agencies helping ill or disabled people at home it acknowledges that this care is palliative. Finally, it differentiates this service from those offering domestic help.

Community palliative care services caring for people at home are sometimes termed 'domiciliary services'.

Day hospice   The term describes a facility for patients under care in the community, who are brought for a few hours each week to a centre, often attached to a hospice/palliative care unit. There they receive clinical care and usually have the opportunity to see a specialist nurse or doctor or social worker, do physiotherapy, occupational and art therapy, and enjoy the company of others in a similar situation to themselves.

It should not be confused with 'Day centre', a term more usually reserved for facilities run by the Social Services in the UK for the elderly, frail and handicapped.

Day care   This term describes care given to patients attending a hospital/hospice/palliative care unit on a day basis rather than having to be admitted for such care. For example, there is day care surgery, day care oncology, day care investigations, day care cardiac catheterization, amongst others.

Complementary therapies   These are treatments which, while not part of traditional, mainstream medicine, nevertheless complement that care. Examples of complementary therapies sometimes offered in palliative care services include hypnotherapy, aromatherapy, homeopathy, and therapeutic massage.

Homemaker   The person whose prime responsibility is to care for the home and the children. The term must not be confused with what in the UK is known as a 'Home Help'—someone employed by a statutory or private agency to shop, cook, and do domestic work for those unable to do so for themselves.

Hospice   As explained in Chapter 1, a 'hospice' and a 'palliative care service' are the same thing. 'Hospice' is the word better known by the general public whilst 'palliative care' is the term adopted by health care professionals because it describes the work done in such a service. In the USA 'hospice' is more usually used to describe the philosophy of care rather than the building or service where it is provided.

Matron   This is the title which might return to common use. It is synonymous with chief nurse, nursing director, head of nursing, director of nursing.

Medical centre   In the UK a medical centre is usually the 'surgery' where prime health care is provided by general practitioners, community nurses, and professionals allied to medicine. In this book, it is the term applied in Australia to a hospital.

Non-malignant diseases   This term embraces the many diseases that are eventually fatal and which need palliative care but which are not related to cancer or other 'malignant' diseases. Examples of non-malignant diseases encountered in palliative care units are end-stage cardiac and respiratory diseases, renal disease, AIDS, and many of the rare incurable conditions afflicting children.

Palliative medicine   There are many definitions of palliative 'care' (the term used when describing the care given by nurses or the palliation team as a whole) and palliative 'medicine' (the term used when describing the care given by doctors). Because some definitions strive to include every aspect of this care they are excessively long. The most succinct is probably: *Palliative medicine is the care of people with active, progressive and far-advanced illness and a short life expectancy, for whom the focus of care is the quality of life.*

Pastoral care worker   This somewhat cumbersome term describes anyone, ordained or not ordained, who caters to the spiritual and religious needs of patients and families. It was coined to avoid terms associated with specific religions or denominations. Titles used range from chaplain and padre to pastoral assistant.

Professions allied to medicine (PAMs)   Included in this term are occupational therapy, physiotherapy, music therapy, art therapy, drama therapy, stoma therapy, dietetics and nutrition, clinical pharmacy, clinical psychology, and complementary therapy.

Specialist palliative care   This is palliative care provided by a professional—doctor, nurse, pharmacist, pastoral care worker—who is accredited as a specialist by their professional body, having undertaken requisite advanced professional training in palliative care. By early 2002, it was a recognized specialty in the UK, Australia, New Zealand, Hong Kong, Sweden, and Romania.

Tertiary referral teaching hospital   Hospitals where undergraduate and postgraduate doctors and nurses are trained are termed 'teaching hospitals'. Most have highly specialized facilities for patients who have been referred by their primary care doctors (GPs) to hospitals and then been referred on again to these specialist centres, hence the term 'tertiary referral'.

Voluntary Service Manager (VSM)   This is the preferred title used in this book for the person more traditionally called the Volunteer Co-ordinator or Co-ordinator of Volunteers.

Index